the DOCTOR'S DIET COOKBOOK

Tasty Meals

for a Lifetime of Vibrant Health
and Weight Loss Maintenance

TRAVIS STORK, M.D.

with Leda Scheintaub

MEDICAL DISCLAIMER

This publication, including the recipes contained herein, is intended to provide helpful and informative material. It is not intended to diagnose, treat, cure, or prevent any health problem or condition, nor is it intended to replace the advice of a physician or dietician. No action should be taken solely on the contents of this book. Always consult your physician, dietician, or qualified health-care professional on any matters regarding your health and before adopting any suggestions or utilizing any recipes in this book or drawing inferences therefrom. Before utilizing any recipes you should always consider possible allergies and allergic reactions to each of the ingredients mentioned in the recipes contained herein.

Be sure to see your own health-care provider before starting *The Doctor's Diet*, initiating an exercise program, or utilizing any recipes contained herein, especially if you have cardiovascular disease, diabetes, or any other health condition.

The Doctor's Diet is not designed for women who are pregnant or breastfeeding. Consult with your obstetrician, your baby's pediatrician, or other qualified health-care professionals on the best nutrition choices during pregnancy and lactation.

The author and publisher specifically disclaim all responsibility for any liability, loss, or risk, personal or otherwise, that is incurred as a consequence, directly or indirectly, from the use or application of any contents of this book.

Any and all product names referenced within this book are the trademarks of their respective owners. None of these owners have sponsored, authorized, endorsed, or approved this book. Always read all information provided by the manufacturers' product labels before using their products. The author and publisher are not responsible for claims made by manufacturers. The statements made in this book have not been evaluated by the US Food and Drug Administration.

This book is dedicated to everyone who has decided to live healthier by making food your medicine. In particular, readers of *The Doctor's Diet* and viewers of *The Doctors* asked for more healthy recipe options, so this is for you!

Acknowledgments

I want to thank first and foremost Leda Scheintaub for her creativity and commitment to this project. I also want to extend a special thank-you to Lisa Clark for her dedication to always getting things right. Thanks to Jon Ford, Ashlee Gagui, and Stuart Smith, as well as to Patricia Austin, Denise McDermott, Radha Newsom, and Gabriel Weiss, for their creative input. And thanks to Jay McGraw, Andrea McKinnon, Joey Carson, and the entire team at Bird Street Books for your continued support!

Contents

Introduction: Falling in Love with Healthy Foods   1

Breakfast   11

Any Berry Smoothie   12

Tropical Fruit Smoothie   14

It's Easy Being Green Smoothie   16

Greek Yogurt Bowl 10 Simple Ways   18

Maple Walnut Granola   20

Chia Seed Cereal   22

Quinoa Porridge   24

10 Recipes to Jazz Up Your Oatmeal   26

Two-Minute Egg DocMuffin   27

Perfectly Scrambled Eggs, with 10 Simple Ways to Serve Them   28

Huevos Rancheros Scramble   30

Poached Egg Perfection, with 10 Ways to Dress Them   32

Shortcut Poached Eggs in Simmering Tomato Sauce   34

Avocado Breakfast Boat   35

Buckwheat Pancakes   37

Savory Pancakes   39

Dips, Spreads, Salsas, and Sauces   41

Southwestern-Style Black Bean Dip   42

Zucchini Hummus   44

Pumpkin Seed Salsa   45

Mint and Black Pepper Greek Yogurt Cheese or Dip   47

The New Pesto   49

Simply Tomato Salsa   50

    Tomato Salsa from Scratch   50

    Tomato Salsa in a Pinch   51

Green Salsa   52

Puttanesca Salsa   53

Corn and Red Onion Salsa   54

Simply Tomato Sauce   56

Instant Guacamole   58

Classic Guacamole   59

Six Simple Ways to Jazz up Your Guacamole   60

16 Sandwich Solutions   61

Soups   63

Cool Cucumber Soup   64

Chilled Avocado and Herb Soup   66

Sweet Carrot Ginger Soup   67

Beet and Mushroom Barley Soup   69

Red Lentil Soup   72

"Not Just Chicken" Chicken Soup   74

Salads   77

Everyday Green Salad All Dressed Up   78

    No Sweat Vinaigrette   80

    Mustard Vinaigrette   81

    Lemon Yogurt Dressing   82

    Asian Sesame Dressing   83

Very Berry Arugula Salad   84

Mighty Green Salad   86

Cucumber Caprese Salad   88

The New Cobb Salad   89

Summer Squash Ribbon Salad   91

Sweet and Tangy Kale Salad   92

"More Than Tuna" Tuna Salad   94

Veggie-Full Sides — 97

Roasted Vegetables 101	104
Anytime Vegetables: A Simple Side-Dish Solution	101
Leafy Greens Made Easy	102
Green Beans with Toasted Coconut	104
Brussels Sprouts Confetti	105
Garlicky Butternut Squash Mash	106
Cauliflower Steak	107
Nudels	109

Whole-Grain Sides — 111

Basic Brown Rice	112
Brown Rice with Asparagus, Peas, and Toasted Almonds	113
Basic Buckwheat	114
Protein-Packed Buckwheat	115
Basic Millet	116
The Sweet Side of Millet	117
Basic Quinoa	118
Quinoa Tabbouleh	119
Basic Whole-Wheat Couscous	120
Zesty Couscous with Summer Squash	121

Mains — 123

No-Fry Falafel	125
Summer Sesame Noodles	128
The New Alfredo	130
Lime-Drenched Pork Salad	132
Festive Fish Tacos	134
Shrimp in Carrot Sauce	136
Shrimp Fra Diavolo	138
Seared Scallops Perfected	140
Fish Fillets Three Simple Ways	142

Poached Salmon Perfected   145

Spinach Curry with Chickpeas   146

Chicken Curry   148

Spicy Chicken Stew   150

Crispy Roasted Chicken   152

Chicken Stock   154

Getting Creative with Chicken Salad   156

    Orange, Fennel, and Rosemary Chicken Salad   156

    Deconstructed Pesto Chicken Salad   157

    Broccoli Chicken Salad   158

Super-Quick Tuna Melt   159

Quicksadillas   160

Mexi Chicken Bowl   162

Chunky Chili   163

Instant Meatballs with Yogurt Sauce   165

Beef and Broccoli Stir-Fry   167

Very Veggie Burgers   169

Veggie Burger on the Go   172

Perfectly Seared Steak   173

The New Comfort Food   175

Nachos   176

Cream of Tomato Soup   178

Creamed Spinach   180

Pizza   182

    Broccoli and Mushrooms with Cauliflower Cheese Sauce   185

    Pesto, Roasted Red Peppers, and Yellow Cherry Tomatoes   185

    Arugula, Fig, and Goat Cheese Pizza   186

Quick Fix Spinach Lasagna   187

The New Classic Burger   189

Zucchini Fries   191

Sweet Potato Fries   192

Doctor Mac and Cheese 193

Eggplant Parmesan 195

Super-Crisp Chicken Wings 197

Oven-Fried Chicken 199

Spaghetti and Meatballs 201

Snacks 203

Chickpea Crunch 205

Crispy Kale Chips 206

Sweet Potato Chips 208

Toasted Nuts 101 209

Chili-Toasted Pumpkin Seeds 210

Power Bites 212

Sweet Treats 215

Peaches and Cream 216

Sliced Apples with Honey 228

Dark Chocolate Mousse 218

Light and Airy Mousse with Cherries 219

Banana Pudding 221

Peanut Butter Bliss 222

Crispy Rice Treats 224

Nuts for Brownies 226

Raspberry Almond Thumbprint Cookies 228

Frozen Lime Cheesecake Bites 230

Berry Vanilla Granita 233

Frozen Yogurt Pops 235

Tropical Chocolate Ice Cream 236

Introduction:
Falling in Love with Healthy Foods

Congratulations! By picking up this book you are taking your daily meals—and your health—into your own hands. A simple but powerful action.

Many of you have arrived at your goal weight or close to it by following the weight-loss plans I shared in *The Doctor's Diet*. First came STAT, a 14-day jump-start plan to lose weight immediately, followed by RESTORE, a second 14-day plan to keep the pounds coming off while broadening your range of eating options. Along the way you learned my 10 Food Prescriptions for optimal health, the backbone of *The Doctor's Diet* and a blueprint for healthy eating for life (see the sidebar to recap, and refer to *The Doctor's Diet* for all the details). If you followed *The Doctor's Diet*, you've faced your weight emergency head-on and have made major shifts in your diet. And you've learned how delicious healthy eating can be. Amazing accomplishment!

This book begins where *The Doctor's Diet* ended, with the MAINTAIN Plan. It provides recipes and tips to help you keep off the pounds you worked so hard to lose while retaining all those health benefits you've gained. MAINTAIN is your launchpad to a

Healthy Eating for Life

The Doctor's Diet 10 Life-Saving Food Prescriptions:

1. Eat with Your Mind
2. Put Protein to Work for You
3. Choose Super-Filling, Fat-Burning Carbohydrates
4. Break Up with Sugar
5. Stop Fearing Fat
6. Fill Your Plate with Vegetables
7. Start Eating Fruit Again
8. Go Nuts Over Nuts
9. Fall in Love with Legumes
10. Go for Yogurt

See *The Doctor's Diet* for a complete discussion of my Food Prescriptions.

lifetime of good health, and the cookbook you're holding in your hands is your support system, your helping hand in the kitchen to encourage you to be creative while staying the course.

It's deliciously simple: the hundred-plus easy-to-make recipes that follow will give you the confidence to cook like you've never cooked before, all while nourishing your body, satisfying your taste buds, and keeping the pounds off, no counting calories required! I'll be right there beside you with helpful hints and guidance every step of the way, and through my "food as medicine" approach you'll learn a lot about the healing properties of food so you can continue to eat your way to perfect health. *The Doctor's Diet* and this cookbook are about a diet—not a diet that you fall off of or get back on, but simply a way of eating for the rest of your long, healthy life. In fact, it's how I eat every single day.

Let Food Be Your Medicine

This inspiration from the father of medicine, Hippocrates, dates back to ancient Greece and is every bit as relevant today. These are words I live by in both my practice and in every recipe in this book; I truly believe that the building blocks of good health are the building blocks of satiety, making this a medicine that's sure to go down easy!

My promise to you is that once you experience this transformative way of eating, you'll naturally gravitate toward healthy foods and effortlessly pass on unhealthy choices. That's because there's no deprivation, no charts or checklists to sit down with, just real food to enjoy, with none of your favorites left behind.

If you love eggs for breakfast, no problem; I'll share with you tips for perfect scrambled and poached eggs every time, with multiple variations to mix up your serving options. If you're not yet a fan of salad, I'll teach you how to make a truly tasty salad, and I'll share with you countless ways to expand your love for veggies. I'll show you how to make a perfect pot of brown rice and widen your whole-grain options to quinoa, buckwheat, millet, and whole-wheat couscous. You'll find no skimpy "diet" food in my mains; what you will find is steak, shrimp, and a variety of globally inspired dishes, all satisfying and full of flavor.

Even favorite comfort foods such as nachos, mac and cheese, and wings are included, and pizza is no longer just pizza, but a veggie delivery system! In my STAT and RESTORE plans, we broke up with sugar, but now dessert is back; I'll show you how even dessert can be medicine when it's based on whole grains, protein, and unrefined sweeteners.

It's a new world of eating, and the adventure starts now! See the sidebar for a review of my MAINTAIN strategies to keep up the motivation (a more detailed version appears in *The Doctor's Diet*).

The Doctor's Diet MAINTAIN Strategies

MAINTAIN Strategy #1: Acknowledge Your Amazing Accomplishments

Even if you're just getting started, you've made some major changes in your health. I am so proud of you! Take some time out every now and then to appreciate that you have now made health your hobby.

MAINTAIN Strategy #2: Be Carb-Smart

See page 5 for the specifics on my Carb-Flex approach.

MAINTAIN Strategy #3: Eat a Wide Variety of Foods

The world of healthy and delicious whole foods is yours to explore. Experiment and try new foods; if you don't like one, go on to the next. Never stop being creative, and don't forget to use herbs and spices in your cooking to give your dishes maximum flavor.

MAINTAIN Strategy #4: Re-create Your Craving Foods

I'd never ask you to give up your favorite foods, be it pizza, eggplant Parmesan, fries, or brownies. What I will ask you to do is turn them into healthy foods. In fact, I've devoted a whole chapter, The New Comfort Food (pages 175 to 202), to this task.

MAINTAIN Strategy #5: Work Off Your Splurges

We're all human, and an occasional splurge is inevitable, even encouraged. No problem—just get right back on the healthy eating track and work those extra calories off with some additional exercise.

MAINTAIN Strategy #6: Weigh Yourself Once a Week

Don't become numbers obsessed, but check in regularly, and if you've gone up a little bit, cut back on the carbs for a while; if the number has crept up by five pounds or more, go back and follow the STAT Plan for a week or two. If you're just three pounds above your goal weight, try returning to RESTORE for a week to get back on track.

MAINTAIN Strategy #7: Monitor Your Health

In addition to checking in with your weight, pay attention to how you feel while you exercise, monitor your blood pressure and anything else your doctor recommends, and don't fall behind in your regular checkups.

MAINTAIN Strategy #8: Move, Move, Move!

Exercise is the closest thing we have to a miracle for preventing the health disasters that send millions of people to the ER every year. The best exercise is one that you love and that works for your body, be it walking, jogging, biking, swimming, skiing, or anything else. My recommendation is to exercise for 30 to 60 minutes most days of the week at an intensity that makes your heart rate go up.

Tasty Meals for a Lifetime of Weight-Loss Maintenance

You're going to love my approach to cooking; no hard-and-fast rules, no formulas to follow except to enjoy food as your medicine every time you sit down to enjoy a meal. It's all about flexibility!

As I mentioned above, you don't need to count calories but, depending on how active you are on a particular day, week, or month, you can make adjustments in terms of portions, carbs, or sweets as you go. My recipes are endlessly adaptable; ultimately I want you to be able to fill in the blanks to create your own healthy meals that you love and always look forward to. Here are some things to keep in mind as you work your way through the recipes.

The Carb-Flex Approach

I introduced this concept in *The Doctor's Diet*; here's how it works: You use your activity levels to guide your carbohydrate amounts. Everyone eats sensible amounts of the healthiest carbohydrates—carbs from vegetables, fruits, legumes, and whole grains, while we minimize simple carbs—sugars and refined grains such as white bread and pasta. Then, if you're going for a nice long run or bicycle ride today, some extra complex carbs might be in order. But if tomorrow it's one meeting after the next with barely time to get up from your desk, you'll go lighter on the complex carbs and favor Anytime Vegetables (see the list on page 101). I do not support super-low-carb diets as a silver bullet for long-term weight loss because they are too restrictive, but I do favor lower carb *days* for when we aren't in a position to burn off those carbs as fuel. My recipes reflect this approach, letting you choose your whole-grain portions from small to large or no-thanks-I'll-pass for any given meal.

The Skinny on Fat

Just as I'm suggesting you choose your carbs based on your level of activity, likewise you can choose the amount of oil you use in a recipe and the level of fat contained in your milk, yogurt, or other dairy, whether it's low-fat or whole, depending on what your calorie goals are on any particular day.

Keep in mind that fat is an essential nutrient needed by every single cell for proper bodily and brain function. Extra-virgin olive oil is one of a few beneficial unsaturated fats you'll see used throughout the book as a go-to healthy option. Conversely, we know that trans fats, in particular hydrogenated and partially hydrogenated oils, are directly implicated in heart disease and should be avoided as much as possible.

But what about saturated fats? Well, a recent large-scale study is changing the way many of us think about saturated fat. This study, a 2014 meta-analysis published in the *American Journal of Clinical Nutrition*, pooled together data from 21 unique studies that included close to 350,000 people, about 11,000 of whom developed cardiovascular disease, tracked them for an average of 14 years, and found no relationship between the intake of saturated fat and the incidence of heart disease or stroke. This new information is worthy of further exploration and there is much left to learn, but given these new findings, don't be surprised if you see a recipe offering the option of a little added butter, full-fat dairy, or cheese in this cookbook. That doesn't mean we know with certainty how these foods play into our overall health but as the research continues, I personally am going to do what I always do whenever there is uncertainty in medical research. I return to my one guiding mantra: everything in balance and moderation.

To Salt or Not

The small amount of salt included in my recipes isn't there to make your food salty but to bring out the natural flavors of the food. Hopefully you've already cut your salt intake enormously by clearing overly processed foods out of your diet, so don't worry about using modest amounts in your recipes. And from there, load up on flavor from the world of herbs, spices, and other seasonings. If your doctor has told you that you are salt-sensitive or have sodium-sensitive hypertension, keep your salt intake at the lowest levels. And don't forget to taste your food before adding more salt.

Options for Vegetarians, Vegans, and the Gluten-Free

The Doctor's Diet Cookbook is adaptable to just about any diet, with many recipes that are naturally vegetarian, vegan, or gluten-free or easily alterable with a variety of options offered. The choice is up to you!

Helping Hands

Throughout the book you'll find a series of recurring sidebars with information on the nutritional and healing properties of foods. Also included are these helpful features:

❖ **Step It Up:** Variations to take your cooking up a notch, when you're up for a little something extra.

❖ **Make It a Meal:** Tips on how to take a salad, side, grain, or other dish and turn it into a complete meal.

- ❖ **Time-saver:** Shortcuts on cutting time without sacrificing taste.
- ❖ **Make Ahead:** Tips on advance planning.
- ❖ **Add Veggies!:** Effortless ways of getting more greens and other vegetables into your dishes.
- ❖ **Label 411:** A mini buyer's guide to supermarket foods and how to read a label (reading the ingredients is the only way to know what's really in your food).
- ❖ ***Dr. T's Gourmet on the Go:*** These recipes are marked with the ⟨Dr. T's Gourmet on the Go⟩ icon; they are the quickest and simplest recipes in the book, your go-to recipes when time is most precious.
- ❖ **On the Simple Side:** These recipes are marked with the ⓢ icon ; they require very few and easy-to-find ingredients and only the most basic of kitchen skills, but do call for just a little more hands-on time than *Dr. T's Gourmet on the Go* recipes. The best part? Even though these dishes are pretty simple to put together, you'll be rewarded with a super-healthy, scrumptious meal.
- ❖ **For the More Adventurous:** These recipes are marked with the Ⓐ icon; try them when you're looking to expand your horizons or take your cooking to the next level.

Dr. T's Gourmet on the Go Recipes

There's no crime in taking shortcuts when it comes to healthy eating—precooked ingredients, using the microwave—it happens sometimes, and in my super-busy life in which I'm crunched for time almost all the time, it happens *a lot!* I get it, and I want you to know you're covered. Just check out these six recipes—Egg DocMuffin (page 27), Quicksadillas (page 160), Quick Fix Spinach Lasagna (page 187), Super-Quick Tuna Melt (page 159), Mexi Chicken Bowl (page 162), and Veggie Burger on the Go (page 172)—for some ideas for lunch or dinner you can have in your hands in just a couple of minutes.

When you're planning for the week, consider making a big pot of whole grains to last you several days (or freeze for longer storage) and double up on mains for leftovers to come home to. Shortcuts such as squeezing a few lemons or limes or chopping a whole lot of garlic or ginger and jarring them (or buying bottles of chopped garlic or ginger) will save you so much time when it comes time to putting together a meal.

Discerning Ingredients

Fill your kitchen with a healthy variety of whole grains, veggies, proteins, and healthy snack options and you've got a kitchen for a very long lifetime!

Whole Grains

Whole grains are a backbone ingredient; I've devoted an entire chapter to them, with basic and stepped-up versions of brown rice, buckwheat, millet, quinoa, and whole-wheat couscous. Enjoy whole grains as part of a balanced diet according to the Carb-Flex approach I've outlined on page 5.

Vegetables

Anytime is a good time to add more veggies to your meals or snacks, perhaps with guacamole, hummus, black bean dip, or any of the dips you'll find on pages 41 to 62. See the list of Anytime Vegetables on page 101; there's really no limit on these veggies—more is good!

Fruit

Fresh fruit is perfect snack material and part of a healthy breakfast. There's no need to worry about overindulging on fruit when you're happy with your weight; fiber-filled fruit is satisfying and doesn't trigger the cravings that come from eating sugary processed foods. No-sugar-added dried fruit is fine in moderation; I prefer to avoid fruit juices and save my extra sugar calories for dessert.

Protein

Whether you're vegetarian or a meat eater or somewhere in between, protein is an important part of every meal, be it from eggs, yogurt, beans, chickpeas, lentils, nuts, seeds, fish, poultry, beef, or pork. Going for free-range and/or grass-fed meats whenever possible is a health-positive choice, as evidence points to higher levels of omega-3 fatty acids in grass-fed meat, potentially making meat a healthier food for your heart (see more on this on page 168). Protein is important in snacking, too, as a smart snack contains protein to keep your hunger satisfied until your next meal.

Oils/Fats

Extra-virgin olive oil is a favorite, as it's heart-healthy, affordable, and available at any supermarket. Other oils such as coconut oil (see page 232) and any made from a nut, seed, or fruit, be it sunflower, avocado, or walnut oil, are worth exploring, and just a little butter adds a lot of flavor to any dish. Just make sure the oil you choose is unrefined, and always avoid hydrogenated and partially hydrogenated oils and trans fats. Fat adds a feeling of satisfaction, so make fat your ally by choosing wisely!

Sweets

Our brains are hardwired to find sweet foods attractive, making any diet that excludes dessert doomed to failure for many people. By favoring desserts containing protein, whole grains, and unrefined sweeteners such as honey and maple syrup, you'll feel satisfied and manage your sugar cravings. Trust me, you won't miss the refined sugar when you've got protein-rich brownies (page 226), crispy rice treats (page 224), chocolate mousse (page 218) and more to choose from!

Remember, you can be healthy and still love food! And you don't have to be a chef to make healthy food really quickly; *The Doctor's Diet Cookbook* will get you feeling like a pro in the kitchen in no time. This is where the fun starts, with food as your medicine in every mouthwatering bite you take. Now let's get cooking!

A Gentle Reminder

Lest you forget how high the stakes are, let's review the statistics. Two out of three Americans are overweight or obese, and more people die of weight-related health complications than car accidents, drug abuse, smoking, and gun violence combined. Obesity is an epidemic that's cost countless lives. I've seen it firsthand in the ER; the majority of patients are often not there because of trauma or accidents but because of their diets. As a doctor, it's my duty to preserve life to the best of my ability. This was my motivation behind writing *The Doctor's Diet,* and this cookbook is designed to keep you at that healthy place. How? By enjoying a wide variety of healthy and tasty meals. And if at any point you've found you've gained a few pounds, the weight-loss principles of STAT and RESTORE from *The Doctor's Diet* are always there to return to.

A Cookbook And So Much More

The mission of *The Doctor's Diet Cookbook* is to fill your kitchen with easy-to-make healthy meals, snacks, and treats for a lifetime of vibrant health and weight loss maintenance. But it's more than just a cookbook. The pages that follow also contain a wealth of valuable nutritional information and fun facts about the foods you're enjoying, guidance on selecting the best quality food from the supermarket, cooking tips, and time-saver techniques to continue to fuel your passion for healthy eating. In addition to picking and choosing recipes from the book, I invite you to grab a healthy snack, kick back, and spend some time flipping through the pages for the sheer enjoyment of it.

Breakfast

I'm a firm believer in breakfast, but most mornings I have just a few precious minutes to dedicate to the most important meal of the day. Luckily, breakfast also happens to be the *easiest* meal of the day, and it can be the most dynamic meal too, as there's no end to the variety of dishes you can make really quickly, from smoothies to scrambles to yogurt bowls and pancakes. In *The Doctor's Diet* I started you off with a handful of quick and easy breakfast recipes, and with this cookbook we're going to expand our horizons (the egg baked in avocado is a must-try!) and get even more creative in the kitchen (chickpea pancakes anyone?), all while keeping time in check.

When it's eggs for breakfast, I think of adding as many Anytime Vegetables (page 101) as possible—why not throw in some spinach or red peppers or onions for variety? If I'm going with a smoothie, my strategy is to see how many fruits or vegetables I can get into the blender, and my cereal bowl is rarely naked but almost always topped with blueberries, raspberries, or whatever fruit's in season.

Your breakfast has failed you if you're hungry an hour later (though there's nothing wrong with a healthy, preferably protein-filled midmorning snack to tide you over to lunch), so this is not the place to cut calorie corners. And if you're bored with your choices, it's another breakfast failure, but there's no chance of that happening here—with 10 variations just on scrambled and poached eggs, a trio of satisfying smoothies, and multiple ways to dress up a simple bowl of cereal just for starters. Let food be your (tasty) medicine from the minute you start your day!

Any Berry Smoothie

SERVES 1

Statistics show that people who eat a good breakfast are trimmer and healthier than those who don't, and you don't need a doctor to tell you you'll have more mental and physical energy to dedicate to your day when you start out with a balanced breakfast.

But breakfast doesn't always have to be a sit-down, fork-in-hand affair. For those days, let your smoothie be your solution—it's an excellent breakfast for the most hurried of mornings, something substantial you can make in less time than it takes to pass through the drive-thru window!

This smoothie calls for baby spinach, but if you happen to have kale in the fridge, go for the kale (remove the tough stems first). Any berry you have on hand is the right berry for this smoothie; go ahead and mix and match, such as raspberries and blueberries or strawberries and cherries, or use a single variety. And if you're low on berries, supplement with peaches, plums, pineapple, banana—anything goes!

+ 1/2 cup water, plus more if needed
+ 1/2 cup plain Greek yogurt
+ 1 cup baby spinach (optional)
+ 1 teaspoon honey or pure maple syrup (optional)
+ 1 cup frozen berries
+ *Optional boosts:* 1 tablespoon flaxseed or chia seeds, 1 scoop protein powder, 1/2 tablespoon all-natural no-sugar-added almond butter

1. Combine all the ingredients in a blender, starting with the water and ending with the berries for easiest blending, and blend, starting on low speed and finishing on high speed until smooth, adding more water if the smoothie is too thick.

2. Pour into a glass and serve immediately.

Variation:

Dairy-Free Any Berry Smoothie: Substitute 1/2 cup coconut milk or nut or other nondairy milk in the carton, or 1/4 cup unsweetened canned coconut milk (not cream of coconut) mixed with 1/4 cup water for the yogurt.

Smoothies vs. Juices

Although fresh-pressed fruit and veggie juices can be filled with nutrients, they are often a concentrated source of sugar and calories as well. Whole smoothies include the fibrous pulp, which contains nutrients and reins in the sugar, allowing it to be digested slowly over time instead of all at once and thereby avoiding spikes in blood sugar that can lead to cravings for more sugar. This fiber is crucial for the digestive system, promoting bowel regularity (how many cookbooks have you read that mention that?!) and feeding beneficial gut bacteria. Many bottled juices that you buy from the shelf really aren't all they're cracked up to be; much of the nutrition has been lost from refinement, and while they are a step up from soda and other processed beverages, they often amount to dessert in a glass.

Tropical Fruit Smoothie

SERVES 1

Start with some yogurt and fruit and your smoothie is guaranteed to be a good one; there's no need to adhere to a specific recipe by the letter. Be adventurous, have fun, and use what's in season or already in the fridge so no fruit or veggie is wasted. There are as many smoothie recipes as there are smoothie makers. And don't worry about overloading on fruit; your body will know when you've had your fill of healthy foods (as opposed to sugary junk food calories, which actually can make you hungrier). What a satisfying feeling!

+ 1/2 cup water
+ 1/2 cup plain Greek yogurt
+ 1/2 banana, broken into chunks (freeze the banana for extra creaminess)
+ 3/4 cup frozen pineapple or mango chunks
+ *Optional boosts:* 1 tablespoon flaxseed or chia seeds, 1 scoop protein powder, 1/2 tablespoon all-natural no-sugar-added almond butter

Step It Up!
Substitute coconut water for the plain water (see page 13).

1. Combine all the ingredients in a blender, starting with the water and ending with the fruit for easiest blending, and blend, starting on low speed and finishing on high speed, until smooth, adding more water if the smoothie is too thick.
2. Pour into a glass and serve immediately.

 Time-saver: Use store-bought frozen mixed tropical fruit chunks.

Protein Powder Pitfalls

Supplementing with protein powder can be a convenient way of getting in a blast of protein. When I was younger and started lifting weights, I used protein powder all the time to help build lean muscle mass. Now I'm so careful about getting protein into every meal that I rarely use it, and if you've been following the principles of healthy eating outlined in *The Doctor's Diet*, you probably won't be turning to it regularly. But there are instances when it comes in handy; for example, if you're skipping the eggs today in favor of a smoothie or have a big workout planned, adding a scoop of protein powder may be just what's needed for top performance and recovery.

When shopping for protein powder, look for a short ingredients list and one that includes no natural or artificial sweeteners and flavorings (many are packed with them). Choose organic if possible from a trusted brand, and be aware of protein powder containing soy isolates, a processed form of soy that can be difficult to assimilate. My favorite is pure, no-frills, highly absorbable whey protein with no added flavorings—you'll be adding all the natural flavors you'll ever need with the fruit in the smoothie. Those of you avoiding dairy might want to explore the numerous emerging options, such as pea, hemp, chia, or chlorella protein powders.

Variation:

Dairy-Free Tropical Fruit Smoothie: Substitute 1/2 cup coconut milk or nut or other nondairy milk in the carton, or 1/4 cup unsweetened canned coconut milk (not cream of coconut) mixed with 1/4 cup water for the yogurt.

It's Easy Being Green Smoothie

SERVES 1

This smoothie packs a mean green punch that will have you buzzing with energy all through the morning (and it doubles as an afternoon pick-me-up).

The key to a tasty green smoothie is including a generous amount of lemon juice, as the citrus provides a perky counterpoint to the earthy greens. Use more lemon juice for bitter greens such as kale and less for milder greens such as lettuce. Smoothie newbies might want to start with milder romaine lettuce and work their way up to deep, dark kale, collards, and other hearty greens. Feel free to mix up your greens, and once you get into a smoothie groove, use this recipe as more of a guideline, a launchpad to signature smoothies of your own creation!

For maximum flavor and nutrition, make your smoothies fresh every time. The recipe easily doubles.

+ 1 cup water
+ 1 tablespoon fresh lemon juice, or to taste
+ 1 packed cup torn spinach, lettuce, kale, collard greens, or other leafy greens (tough stems removed from heartier greens)
+ Small handful of fresh mint or cilantro (optional)
+ 1/2 to 1 small ripe banana, broken into pieces, or 1/2 to 1 small apple or pear, cored and chopped
+ Handful of ice cubes
+ *Optional boosts:* 1 tablespoon flaxseed or chia seeds, 1 scoop protein powder, 1/2 tablespoon all-natural no-sugar-added almond butter

How Important Is Organic?

More and more people are becoming concerned with how their food is grown, and organic has become an increasingly popular eating choice. There are many good reasons to favor organic, such as reducing your family's exposure to potentially harmful pesticides and additives and, in the case of dairy and meat, decreasing your intake of excess hormones and antibiotics (especially important for growing children).

For me as an ER doctor, keeping you away from overly processed products and unhealthy fast food is my number-one priority. Going organic is a next step, but it doesn't have to be an all-or-nothing type of choice, as going full-on organic can be pricey and doesn't fit into many budgets. A good in-between measure is favoring organic for produce that is highest in pesticides when conventionally grown, such as fruits and vegetables that have made it on to the Environmental Working Group's Dirty Dozen list. As of this writing the list included apples, strawberries, grapes, celery, peaches, spinach, sweet bell peppers, nectarines (imported), cucumbers, cherry tomatoes, snap peas (imported), and potatoes. See the Environmental Working Group's website, ewg.org, for more information, or download their Dirty Dozen App.

1. In a blender, combine the water, lemon juice, spinach, and mint, if using, and blend, starting on low speed and finishing on high speed, until smooth. Add the banana and ice and blend again, starting on low speed and finishing on high speed, until smooth, and adding more water if the smoothie is too thick.

2. Pour into a glass and serve immediately.

Step It Up!

❖ Add 1 small stalk celery, including leaves, chopped.

❖ Swap in avocado as your fruit to add some healthy fats.

❖ Substitute coconut water for the plain water (see page 13).

Greek Yogurt Bowl 10 Simple Ways

As anyone who has read The Doctor's Diet knows, I love yogurt. I favor Greek yogurt, as it is lower in carbs and sugar than regular yogurt. A cup of plain Greek yogurt is the base for my breakfast bowl, and here are some of my favorite ways to serve it up.

1. Tropical Yogurt Bowl: *Top 1 cup plain Greek yogurt with 1 cut-up kiwi and 1/2 cut-up banana (freeze the other half for the Tropical Fruit Smoothie, page 14). Sprinkle with a handful of chopped unsalted roasted cashews or unsweetened coconut flakes.*

2. Granola Yogurt Parfaits: *Fill a parfait glass with alternating layers of plain Greek yogurt, granola (page 20), and fresh fruit; drizzle with a teaspoon of pure maple syrup if you like.*

3. On-the-Go Fruit Parfaits: *Fill pint-size mason jars with alternating layers of plain Greek yogurt and fruit. Cover and store in the fridge until breakfast time (make it the night before) and enjoy at home or at the office.*

4. Melon Yogurt Bowl: *Use half a cantaloupe as your bowl; fill with 1 cup plain Greek yogurt and top with berries and pumpkin seeds.*

5. Smoothie Yogurt Bowl: *Blend 1 cup plain Greek yogurt with 1 cup frozen berries and a little honey if you like until smooth. Top with toasted nuts (page 209) or granola (page 20).*

A Healthful Bowl of Cereal

Kids like cereal for breakfast, no two ways about it, as do most adults! That's great—cereal can be a quick and healthy breakfast option, but for you hurried parents out there, my advice to you is to build a substantial and satisfying bowl of cereal with my three-part plan of action: 1) choose whole-grain, lower-sugar cereal (see page 23 to learn how); 2) make sure you're getting some protein in the form of plain yogurt or milk, be it dairy milk, coconut milk, or a nut-based milk; and 3) don't forget to finish with fresh fruit. Fruit is where kids can take control of their bowl: let them choose what they like—peaches, kiwis, berries, bananas, or all of the above. Have a selection on hand to please every eater at the table.

6. Peach and Cinnamon Yogurt Bowl: *Top 1 cup plain Greek yogurt with 1 diced peach; finish with a dusting of cinnamon.*

7. Chia Cereal Yogurt Bowl: *Top 1 cup plain Greek yogurt with 1/2 cup of your favorite whole-grain (or bran) boxed cereal (see page 23 on choosing a healthy one) and a sprinkling of chia seeds.*

8. Maple Walnut Yogurt Bowl: *Top 1 cup plain Greek yogurt with a drizzle of pure maple syrup and a handful of toasted walnuts.*

9. Cherry Vanilla Yogurt Bowl: *Mash 1/4 cup frozen defrosted unsweetened cherries along with 1/2 teaspoon vanilla extract into 1 cup plain Greek yogurt.*

10. Savory Avocado Yogurt Bowl: *Remove the pit from 1/2 avocado and top with a dollop of plain Greek yogurt (you won't fit a whole cup in this one); drizzle with extra-virgin olive oil and top with herbs, a pinch of salt, and a little hot sauce if you like.*

Maple Walnut Granola

MAKES ABOUT 10 CUPS

Granola, with its high protein and fiber profile, can be part of a healthy diet, but enjoy it in moderation, as it's a dense and calorie-rich dish, and a little goes a long way. I sometimes sprinkle it onto my yogurt, and it adds crunch to a breakfast bowl parfait (page 18), but it's not something to sit down and eat by the bowlful. Think of it more as a garnish or a flourish than a complete breakfast food.

There's a lot of junk-food granola out there masquerading as healthful breakfast food, whereas this quick mix-and-bake recipe assures your granola is made with health-supportive sweeteners and quality oils and will last you a couple of months. And if homemade isn't an option this week, see below on how to choose a healthful store-bought brand.

+ 8 cups rolled oats (not quick-cooking)
+ 2 cups coarsely chopped walnuts, pecans, peanuts, cashews, or a combination
+ 1 teaspoon ground cinnamon
+ 1/4 teaspoon salt
+ 3/4 cup melted virgin coconut or other oil
+ 2/3 cup pure maple syrup or honey
+ 1 tablespoon pure vanilla extract

 Make Ahead: Make a batch of granola on a Sunday and it will keep you flush in granola for a month or two.

Granola: Fit or Fake?

The average person equates the term *granola* with health food because many of the ingredients in granola are healthful. The reality is that many brands of granola also contain some not-so-healthy ingredients, most notably hydrogenated or otherwise refined oils and refined sugar. In fact, most granola is much higher in sugar than your average supermarket breakfast cereal. Even wholesome-sounding descriptions such as *honey-toasted* or *maple syrup–sweetened* are not above suspicion—plain old white sugar often makes its way into the mix as well, and in large quantities.

When shopping for granola, favor varieties sweetened with honey or maple syrup (and make sure it's *pure* maple syrup). Beware of brands that boast of "low-fat" content, as they often eliminate some of the most healthful ingredients, such as nuts. (FYI: All of the above goes for granola bars as well.) When it comes to granola labels, short and not so sweet is the way to go!

1. Preheat the oven to 300°F.

2. Combine the oats, nuts, cinnamon, and salt in a large bowl. In a medium bowl, whisk together the oil, maple syrup, and vanilla. Pour the oil mixture over the oat mixture and stir well to combine and coat evenly.

3. Spread the oat mixture over two large baking sheets in an even layer. Bake for about 1 hour, stirring every 15 minutes, until the granola is lightly browned and slightly crisp (it will crisp up further as it cools).

4. Turn off the oven and let cool for about 1 hour in the pan, until completely cooled, then pour the granola into a container, cover, and store in the pantry, where it will keep for up to 2 months.

Chia Seed Cereal

SERVES 1

Who would have known that chia seeds (yes, they are what chia pets are made from!) could transform themselves into a creamy, fiber-filled break-fast cereal? While chia seeds are new to many of us, they are becoming increasingly available in supermarkets and can fit easily into any cooking routine. See the sidebar to learn what makes this superfood one you'll want to enjoy often.

+ 3 tablespoons chia seeds
+ 1 cup almond milk or other milk
+ 1 teaspoon pure vanilla extract
+ 1 tablespoon pure maple syrup or honey
+ *Flavoring options:* ground cinnamon, nutmeg, or allspice
+ *Topping options:* sliced apple, pear, banana, or other fruit, plain Greek yogurt
+ *Sweetener options:* splash of pure maple syrup or honey

1. Combine all the ingredients (except the topping options) in a bowl and stir until combined.
2. Cover and let sit for at least 15 minutes or up to overnight in the refrigerator. Alternatively, for a smoother cereal, combine the ingredients in a blender and blend until well combined.

Make Ahead: Combine the cereal ingredients the night before and keep in the refrigerator, where it will be ready for breakfast. The recipe doubles easily for multiple breakfasts throughout the week.

LABEL 411

Breakfast Cereal

Boxed cereal can be a world of extremes, from hard-core twigs to sugary sweet dessert. Cereal can be a healthy, convenient option for breakfast, but read the nutrition label carefully to make sure your cereal is based on a whole grain. A good rule of thumb is to choose a cereal with a whole grain as the first ingredient. If the word *whole* doesn't appear before *grain*, usually the grain is refined (e.g., *wheat* most likely means white flour rather than whole wheat). One caveat to that rule might be bran cereal; bran represents the outer core of a whole grain and it can add a great fiber punch to your breakfast. Give your bowl added flavor and a nutritional boost with seasonal fruit, ground cinnamon, or shaved nuts.

Pass the Chia Seeds Please

The Aztecs believed chia seeds were sacred, and their messengers would carry bags of them on their hips when running hundreds of miles. Chia seeds can absorb about 10 times their weight in water, making them quite hydrating and extremely digestible.

Chia seeds are a great source of complete vegetarian protein. They are rich in calcium, magnesium, and phosphorus, packed with antioxidants, and an amazing source of health-essential fats, with two tablespoons boasting more than 4,000 milligrams of omega-3 fatty acids. (Omega-3s are crucial to the heart, brain, and every system of the body; while there is no agreed-upon daily requirement for these fatty acids, generally it is recommended that we consume 1,500 to 3,000 milligrams daily for optimal health.) They are very versatile in cooking—added to smoothies, breakfast cereal, and puddings, for example—and are available in most natural food stores and some supermarkets.

How to Enjoy Chia Seeds

❖ Sprinkled onto hot or cold cereal
❖ Stirred into yogurt
❖ Blended into smoothies
❖ Mixed into granola
❖ Baked into muffins
❖ Added to pancake batter or sprinkled on top
❖ Added to salad dressing as a thickener
❖ In pudding (see page 221)

23

Quinoa Porridge

SERVES 4

Go beyond oatmeal to nutty, fluffy quinoa and you've effortlessly broadened your breakfast options. Unsweetened, it's a side to eggs in place of toast, or serve traditional porridge style with a drizzle of milk and honey and a little fruit. See page 171 to learn about the health benefits of quinoa.

+ 1 cup quinoa
+ 2½ cups water
+ Pinch of salt
+ 1 cup almond milk, another nondairy milk, or dairy milk, plus more for serving
+ *Flavoring options:* ground cinnamon, nutmeg, or allspice
+ *Topping options:* plain Greek yogurt; sliced apple, pear, banana, or other fruit; walnuts or other nuts or flaxseeds
+ *Sweetener options:* splash of pure maple syrup or honey

1. Rinse the quinoa well in a strainer under cold running water.
2. Combine the quinoa, water, and salt in a medium saucepan. Place over medium heat and bring to a simmer. Reduce the heat, cover, and

Make Ahead: Make a big pot of porridge on a Sunday and microwave by the bowlful for a breakfast any or every day of the week.

cook for 15 minutes. Add the milk, return to a simmer, and cook, covered, for another 10 minutes, or until softened and fluffy.

3. Stir in the flavorings of your choice, spoon into bowls, and serve, with milk poured on top, your choice of toppings, and a splash of maple syrup or honey.

Just the Cold, Hard Flax

Flaxseeds are another great source of omega-3s that have been consumed for thousands of years. Mahatma Gandhi once observed: "Wherever flaxseed becomes a regular food item among the people, there will be better health." As whole seeds, they are harder to digest than chia seeds, so it's best to grind them before using.

Flaxseeds are a rich source of lignans, substances that appear to positively affect hormone-related problems and reduce the risk of various forms of cancer and may also be useful in the treatment of obesity and diabetes. Flax and chia seeds have comparable levels of omega-3s, and both provide an awesome array of minerals. No need to choose just one when you can enjoy them both.

10 Recipes to Jazz Up Your Oatmeal

1. Apple Pie Oats: *Top with chopped apples, walnuts, cinnamon, and a drizzle of pure maple syrup.*

2. Greek Yogurt Oats: *Stir some plain Greek yogurt into your bowl in place of milk.*

3. Choco-Oats: *Sprinkle with a spoonful of unsweetened dark cocoa powder and a drizzle of honey; add a few dark chocolate chips for special occasions.*

4. Pumpkin Pie Oats: *Stir in a spoonful of canned pumpkin puree (not pumpkin pie filling) and dust with pumpkin pie spice or cinnamon, cloves, and nutmeg.*

5. Nutty Banana Oats: *Add sliced banana and a spoonful of all-natural no-sugar-added peanut butter or almond butter.*

6. Apple and Cheddar Oats: *Top with chopped apples, a drizzle of pure maple syrup, and a little grated cheddar cheese.*

7. Very Berry Oats: *Top with any variety of fresh berry or a mixture; if using frozen berries, stir them into the oatmeal as it cooks.*

8. Egg and Herb Oats: *Skip the milk and sweetener and top with a poached egg, some herbs, and a squeeze of Sriracha hot sauce if you like.*

9. Cheese and Avocado Oats: *Top with a little grated cheese, avocado slices, and a drizzle of extra-virgin olive oil.*

10. Trail Mix Oats: *Top with any seeds, such as chia, flax, sesame, or pumpkin seeds, and raisins.*

Two-Minute Egg Egg DocMuffin

SERVES 1

Eggs are not the culprit for our overweight crisis; eggs in moderation are a great breakfast protein option, and this is my favorite way to make them when I've literally got just a couple of minutes to get my a.m. meal together. And did you know that the calorie count of an entire whole-grain English muffin equals that of just one slice of bread? Good to know when your DocMuffin is made-to-go and open-faced isn't an option.

+ Extra-virgin olive oil cooking spray
+ 1 large egg
+ Freshly ground black pepper or ground cayenne
+ Pinch of salt (optional)
+ 1 whole-wheat English muffin or 1 slice whole-grain bread, toasted

Step It Up!
Throw in a handful of spinach before adding the egg.

1. Spray a microwave-safe dish with cooking spray and crack the egg into the dish. Sprinkle with pepper and the salt, if using.

2. Cover and microwave for 1 minute, or until set. Slide the egg onto the English muffin and serve.

Variations:

Avocado-Mustard Egg DocMuffin: Spread a little mustard over the toasted English muffin; slice 1/4 ripe avocado and spread it over the mustard.

Cheese and Egg DocMuffin: Add 1 tablespoon of grated cheese to the bowl after microwaving for the first 30 seconds.

Perfectly Scrambled Eggs,
with 10 Simple Ways to Serve Them

SERVES 1

With these easy instructions, rubbery scrambled eggs are a thing of the past! The key to success is to declare your scramble done when the eggs are just set and still a little moist, as cooking continues a bit after you turn off the heat. A pinch of turmeric deepens the golden color of your scramble and gives your morning meal a hit of anti-inflammatory action.

+ 1 large egg
+ 1 large egg white
+ Small pinch of ground turmeric (optional)
+ Pinch of salt and freshly ground black pepper
+ Extra-virgin olive oil cooking spray or 1 teaspoon butter

1. In a large bowl, beat the egg and egg white with 1 teaspoon water and the turmeric, salt, and pepper until light and foamy.

2. Heat a large skillet over medium heat and spray with cooking spray or melt the butter in it. Add the eggs and don't touch them for about 1 minute, until they begin to set. Then, using a rubber spatula, gently fold the eggs until they still look a tiny bit wet, another minute or so. Then, turn off the heat and fold the eggs a few more times.

3. Place the eggs on a plate. Serve immediately, dressed up any way you like them (see below).

Add Veggies!
Serve veggies alongside or tossed into the eggs as they finish cooking—anything goes (see page 101 for Anytime Vegetables).

No Skillet Scrambled Eggs

Here's a really quick way to prepare Perfectly Scrambled Eggs without a skillet. Spray a deep microwave-safe bowl with cooking spray. Add the eggs, egg whites, turmeric, salt, and pepper and whisk until foamy. Cover and microwave on high for 1 minute, then stir gently with a fork (wear an oven mitt, as the bowl will get hot) so any uncooked egg blends with the cooked egg. Return the eggs to the microwave and microwave in 30-second intervals, stirring each time, until the eggs are almost set, making sure not to overcook them. Remove from the microwave and serve.

10 Ways to Dress Up Your Scrambled Eggs

1. **Herby Scramble:** Stir in generous amounts of herbs: cilantro, basil, parsley, dill, whatever you like.
2. **Rosemary and Cherry Tomato Scramble:** Stir in halved or quartered cherry tomatoes and a sprinkling of minced fresh rosemary or dried rosemary.
3. **Green Eggs and Ham:** Stir some pesto (page 48) into your eggs and serve with a slice of all-natural ham or turkey ham.
4. **Whole-Grain Scramble:** Serve with a whole grain (pages 111 to 122) instead of toast.
5. **Thai-Style Scramble:** Add a little fish sauce (available in the Asian food aisle) and fresh lime juice.
6. **Green Hollandaise Scramble:** Top with Green Hollandaise (page 33).
7. **Breakfast Burrito:** Heat whole-grain tortillas and fill with scrambled eggs; top with a little grated cheese, salsa (pages 50 to 54), and hot sauce and roll it up.
8. **Green Burrito:** Make the breakfast burrito as above, but roll it in a collard green leaf (remove the tough part of the stem first) instead of a tortilla.
9. **Spicy Scramble:** Add some cayenne or hot powdered mustard when you whisk the eggs.
10. **Cheesy Chile Scramble:** Add a light sprinkle of cheese and some sliced jalapeños after cooking (a little bit of cheese goes a long way in flavoring your scramble).

Huevos Rancheros Scramble

SERVES 2

This shortcut version of the Mexican brunch favorite skips the double dose of frying (fried eggs and fried tortillas) you'll find on restaurant menus, making it lighter, healthier, and completely doable any day of the week.

+ Extra-virgin olive oil cooking spray
+ 2 large eggs
+ 2 large egg whites
+ Pinch of ground turmeric (optional)
+ 1/4 teaspoon salt, or to taste
+ 2 corn tortillas (see page 135 on how to choose them), ripped into pieces
+ 1/2 cup Simply Tomato Salsa (page 50) or jarred salsa, slightly warmed
+ 1/4 cup shredded Jack cheese
+ Optional toppings: sliced raw onion, chopped fresh cilantro

1. In a large bowl, beat the egg and egg white with 2 teaspoons water, the turmeric, if using, and the salt until light and foamy. Add the tortillas and let sit for about 10 minutes, until tortillas are slightly softened.

Add Veggies!
Serve on a bed of spinach or mixed greens.

Turmeric: Curry's Secret Weapon

Turmeric is the spice that gives a golden hue to curries; in India this food is also used as medicine for its antioxidant and anti-inflammatory properties. The pigment that gives turmeric its characteristic color, known as curcumin, is responsible for turmeric's healing action, and studies attest to its potency. A comprehensive summary published by James A. Duke, PhD, in the October 2007 issue of *Alternative and Complementary Therapies* reviewed more than 700 individual studies and concluded that turmeric may outperform many pharmaceuticals in the treatment of major debilitating diseases, including Alzheimer's disease, arthritis, and cancer, without toxic side effects. As we are learning with many foods and spices, turmeric may even work in combination with a healthy lifestyle to prevent these conditions.

So spice up your meals with turmeric if you desire—its flavor is mild, making it easy to include a sprinkle in just about any recipe without changing the taste of the food. Add a little to your scramble and you'll never know there's an extra egg white in the mix.

2. Spray a large nonstick skillet with cooking spray and heat it over medium heat. Add the eggs and leave them for about 1 minute, until they begin to set. Then, using a rubber spatula, gently fold the eggs and keep folding them until they still look a tiny bit wet but are completely set, another minute or two.

3. Divide the eggs between 2 plates. Top with the salsa, followed by the cheese and your choice of toppings. Serve immediately.

Poached Egg Perfection,
with 10 Ways to Dress Them

MAKES 2 POACHED EGGS

Once you learn how to poach your eggs to perfection you'll feel like a superstar chef in your very own kitchen. Now every day can be Sunday brunch!

+ 2 large eggs
+ 2 tablespoons white wine vinegar or apple cider vinegar

1. Break the eggs into two separate teacups and line a plate with a paper towel.

2. Fill a wide shallow saucepan about two-thirds full with water. Bring to a boil over high heat and add the vinegar. Reduce the heat to very low so it's just barely simmering.

3. Using the straight end of a wooden spoon, stir to create a whirlpool in the water and gently add the eggs one at a time by lowering the cups directly into the center of the whirlpool and gently tipping in the eggs.

4. Cook until the whites are set and the yolks starts to thicken, about 3 minutes for a soft yolk, about 5 minutes for a hard yolk. Lift the poached eggs out of the water using a slotted spoon and place on the paper towel–lined plate to drain.

Make Ahead: Bump up the number of eggs you poach; as you poach them, slip them into a bowl of ice water to cool, dry them on paper towels, and store in the refrigerator for up to 5 days. Reheat by briefly dropping them into a pot of simmering water. Poach several on Sunday for breakfasts throughout the week.

Poached Eggs: 10 Ways to Dress Them

1. **Turkish-Style Poached Eggs:** Spread a dollop of plain Greek yogurt onto a plate; top with a poached egg and finish with a drizzle of extra-virgin olive oil and a sprinkle of paprika and mint.

2. **Anytime Poached Eggs:** Serve over an Anytime Vegetable (page 101).

3. **Naked Poached Eggs:** Serve solo over whole-grain toast.

4. **Poached Eggs with Green Hollandaise:** In a blender or food processor, combine the flesh of 1/2 small avocado, 1 tablespoon fresh lemon juice, and 6 tablespoons water and blend until smooth and light in texture, about 2 minutes, scraping down the sides of the machine once or twice and adding more water if needed to thin it out. With the machine running, slowly drizzle in 1 tablespoon extra-virgin olive oil and blend until incorporated. Season with salt and pepper and serve over your poached eggs.

5. **Pesto Poached Eggs:** Top with pesto (page 48).

6. **Savory Pancake with Poached Egg:** Serve over a Savory Pancake (page 39) with your choice of toppings, such as hot sauce and fresh herbs.

7. **Florentine-Style Poached Eggs:** Heat leftover Creamed Spinach (page 180) and spread it over whole-grain toast; top with a poached egg.

8. **Salsa Poached Eggs:** Top with Green Salsa (page 52), Simply Tomato Salsa (page 50), or a jarred tomato salsa; serve over fresh tomato slices.

9. **Poached Egg over Hummus:** Spread Zucchini Hummus (page 44), Pumpkin Seed Salsa (page 45), or an all-natural store-bought hummus over whole-grain toast (or try Smoky Black Bean Dip, page 43, or guacamole, page 59); top with a poached egg.

10. **Dinner for Breakfast (or Breakfast for Dinner):** Reheat leftovers from last night's dinner and top with a poached egg.

Shortcut Poached Eggs in Simmering Tomato Sauce

SERVES 2 TO 4

Poaching your eggs couldn't be easier and quicker: just heat up tomato sauce, crack in your eggs, cover, and breakfast is on. Feel free to go beyond tomato sauce and use any sauce or dish you have handy in the fridge, such as last night's leftover quinoa or brown rice or just about anything else to serve as a poaching base.

+ 1½ cups Simply Tomato Sauce (page 56) or low-sodium store-bought tomato sauce
+ 4 large eggs
+ Salt and freshly ground black pepper
+ 2 to 4 slices whole-wheat toast or 1 to 2 cups leftover brown rice or another whole grain (pages 111 to 122)
+ Grated Parmesan cheese (optional)

1. Pour the tomato sauce into a medium skillet, place over medium heat, and bring to a simmer.
2. Crack the eggs directly into the sauce, cover, and cook for about 5 minutes, until the whites are set and the yolks are cooked to your liking. Uncover, season with salt and pepper to taste, and serve the eggs over toast or a whole grain of your choice. Top with a sprinkling of Parmesan if you like.

Add Veggies!
Add a side of Anytime Vegetables (see the list on page 101).

Avocado Breakfast Boat

SERVES 2

Sail into new breakfast territory with this effortless way to enjoy my favorite green fruit. Serve with a spoon for scooping or spread onto toast—you choose. High in protein and fiber, low in carbs, and fun for the whole family!

+ 1 ripe avocado
+ 2 eggs
+ Couple squeezes of lime juice
+ Pinch of salt
+ Sriracha or other hot sauce (optional)
+ Chopped fresh scallions, chives, cilantro, mint, or parsley
+ 1 slice crumbled cooked pork or turkey bacon (optional)
+ 2 slices whole-wheat toast or whole-wheat or corn tortillas (optional)

1. Preheat the oven to 450°F and line a small baking pan with parchment or foil.
2. Cut the avocado in half and remove the pit. If necessary, slice off a sliver of the bottom of the avocado using a serrated knife so it can sit flat. Scoop out a little of the avocado to extend the hole to fit the egg (save the scraps to garnish the finished dish). Place the avocado halves on the prepared baking pan and squeeze a little lime juice over them.

Continues ▶

When You Go for the Bacon . . .

Personally I go with real pork bacon rather than turkey bacon on the rare occasion I eat it. That's because turkey bacon often contains comparable calories, fat, and sodium to pork bacon, so it is not always a healthier choice. And with research coming out questioning the link between saturated fats in meat and heart disease (see page 5), my advice is to eat the type of bacon you enjoy the most—be it pork or turkey—but do so in moderation. A slice or two is all that's needed alongside your eggs, crumbled atop a salad, or nestled into a sandwich for maximum satisfaction. Just remember to read the ingredients list, favoring brands lowest in sodium and free of nitrates or other preservatives and other unnatural additives.

3. Break an egg into a bowl and slide into an avocado half. Repeat with the other avocado half. Don't worry if some of the white spills out as long as the yolk stays intact.

4. Place in the oven and bake for 8 to 10 minutes, until the eggs are set to your liking.

5. Remove from the oven, place on plates, sprinkle with the salt, add another squeeze of lime, and drizzle with hot sauce if you like. Top with the avocado scraps, the scallions, and bacon, if using. Serve with the toast, if including, to scoop up every single bit.

 Time-saver: Bake your boats in a toaster oven.

Buckwheat Pancakes

MAKES ABOUT 16 PANCAKES

Pancakes are a special treat for me, and when I make them they're always whole grain based. Hearty yet light buckwheat gives you the sustenance to get you through the morning without that blood sugar crash often associated with refined flour pancakes, and mashed banana adds natural sweetness and keeps your pancakes moist and light. Poached or scrambled eggs make a perfect protein companion. I'll generally eat one pancake as my breakfast carb, two if I'm planning to be particularly active that day.

Making from-scratch pancakes takes a little extra time, but I think you'll find it well worth the effort, and as a bonus you'll save money by skipping store-bought pancake mix.

To keep batches of pancakes warm, transfer them to a baking sheet in a preheated 200°F oven as you make them.

+ 2 cups milk
+ 1 large egg
+ 1 very ripe banana, sliced
+ 1/2 teaspoon pure vanilla extract
+ 1 cup buckwheat flour
+ 1/2 cup whole-wheat flour
+ 1 tablespoon baking powder
+ Pinch of salt
+ Extra-virgin olive oil cooking spray or butter

Continues ▶

Make Ahead: The batter will keep for up to 3 days; keep it ready for any-morning pancake making.

- *Topping options:* plain Greek yogurt, berries or other fruit, small pats of butter, toasted walnuts or other nuts (page 209), unsweetened dried coconut, dusting of cinnamon or nutmeg
- *Sweetener options:* pure maple syrup or honey

1. In a blender or food processor, combine the milk, egg, banana, and vanilla and blend until smooth. Add the buckwheat and whole-wheat flours, the baking powder, and salt and blend just to combine. Add a little water if the mixture is too thick for pouring.

2. Spray a nonstick skillet or griddle with cooking spray or add a pat of butter to it and heat over medium heat. Ladle in batter, about 1/4 cup for each pancake, and cook on one side until bubbles begin to form on the surface and the pancake is set and lightly browned on the bottom, about 2 minutes. Flip the pancakes and cook on the second side until lightly browned and cooked through, another minute or two.

3. Serve immediately, with your choice of toppings and sweetener.

Variations:

Touch of Heaven Pancakes: Add a few dark chocolate chips (you won't need many for that heavenly effect) to your pancakes just after you pour the batter onto the skillet and cook as above. Drizzle with maple syrup.

Buckwheat Berry Pancakes: Add a scattering of raspberries or blueberries to the pancake batter just after you pour the batter into the pan, before it sets.

Double Banana Buckwheat Pancakes: Arrange banana slices onto the pancake batter just after you pour the batter into the pan, before it sets.

Gluten-Free Buckwheat Pancakes: Substitute almond flour or rice flour for the whole-wheat flour.

Savory Pancakes

MAKES 6 TO 8 PANCAKES

While this may not be for everyone, it definitely takes the cake when it comes to a different kind of pancake. This pancake is lighter yet more substantial than your typical pancake and welcomes generous amounts of vegetables to complete it. It's protein packed and has amazing binding powers without the assistance of eggs, making it a no-fail pancake. The secret is its chickpea flour base; you can find this ingredient in natural food stores, Indian and international groceries, and some supermarkets.

+ 1 cup chickpea flour
+ 1/4 teaspoon onion powder
+ 1/4 teaspoon garlic powder
+ 1/2 teaspoon salt, or to taste
+ 1 cup water
+ 1/2 cup plain yogurt
+ 1/4 teaspoon baking soda
+ Extra-virgin olive oil cooking spray or butter

1. Place the flour in a large bowl and whisk it to break up any lumps. Add the onion powder, garlic powder, and salt and whisk again, then whisk in the water, followed by the yogurt. If you have the time, let the batter sit for 10 minutes or so.

Continues ▶

The Revival of Butter

Butter has been enjoyed for thousands of years by people all over the world, and recent research has suggested that butter, along with the saturated fats found in meat and whole-milk dairy, may not be the culprits in heart disease we once thought them to be (see more on page 5). Studies are ongoing, and I'm not recommending you go on a butter binge, but butter does happen to have a noteworthy nutrition profile: it contains a highly absorbable form of iodine and vitamin A, vitamins E and D, and minerals, including selenium, manganese, chromium, and zinc.

It only takes a small amount of butter to elevate a dish and add an element of satisfaction—and when we're satisfied with our food, we are less prone to overindulge.

So while I still recommend focusing your cooking and eating around fats and oils we know are healthy, like olive oil, I personally believe it's OK to occasionally bring the butter back to the table—as long as you enjoy it in moderation—but pass on the white bread!

2. Just before you are ready to make the pancakes, whisk in the baking soda.

3. Spray a nonstick skillet with cooking spray and heat it over medium heat. Add about 1/3 cup of the batter and tilt the skillet to spread it out to a 5-inch or so pancake. Immediately add about 1/4 cup toppings to the surface of the wet batter and cook until browned on the underside and the top has set, about 2 minutes.

4. Flip the pancake and cook on the other side for another minute or two, until cooked through and browned on the second side. Transfer to a plate and serve.

 Make Ahead: Make the whole batch of pancakes, cool, place in zip-top bags with a square of wax paper between each, and store in the freezer. Thaw and heat them up in the microwave or a toaster oven.

Dips, Spreads, Salsas, and Sauces

This foursome of kitchen staples is just what you need anytime you're looking to enhance an entrée, snack, or sandwich. They'll expand your palate, with herbs and spices creating new taste sensations, all while you enjoy their nutrient-rich profile. They're easy to make, they extend your kitchen options exponentially, and every single ingredient in them is waist and heart healthy! Go light with the chips for dipping and favor Anytime Vegetables—see the list on page 101 for ideas—and consider expanding your options from the standard carrots and bell peppers to less common veggies such as jicama and turnips.

Note: If the thought of making your own spread or sauce from scratch is too much, not to worry! There are many healthy packaged dips, spreads, salsas, and the like on the market. So, if you don't have the time or desire to go DIY in this department, look for store-bought options that are low in sodium and made with extra-virgin olive oil or another healthy oil and contain no preservatives or additives.

Southwestern-Style Black Bean Dip

MAKES ABOUT 1½ CUPS

I'm a huge fan of this dip for the range of flavors it brings with every dip of the chip or carrot stick, and it's equally tasty in a sandwich or as a topping for nachos (page 176). If you have the time, let the dip sit for 30 minutes before serving for the flavors to mingle.

- 1 (15-ounce) can no-salt-added black beans, drained and rinsed
- 1/2 small red onion, chopped
- 2 tablespoons Simply Tomato Salsa (page 50) or jarred salsa (optional)
- 2 garlic cloves, chopped
- 1/2 to 1 small jalapeño chile (optional)
- 1/2 small bunch fresh cilantro, including stems, chopped (save a few leaves for garnish if you like)
- 2 tablespoons fresh lime juice, or to taste
- 2 tablespoons plain Greek yogurt
- 1 teaspoon honey (optional)
- 1 teaspoon ground cumin
- 1/2 teaspoon ground coriander
- 1/4 teaspoon ground cayenne
- 1/2 teaspoon salt, or to taste

 Make Ahead: The dip will keep, covered and refrigerated, for up to 5 days, to have it handy for impromptu snacking throughout the week.

Canned Beans Basics

Canned beans are a great convenience and an invaluable tool for meal building. But watch your labels: favor no-salt-added and preservative-free beans, and look for cans labeled *BPA free*. BPA, or bisphenol A, is a chemical often found in the lining of canned beans, tomatoes, and other foods as well as in certain plastics. It's been in the spotlight for its potentially negative health effects on hormones and the brain, particularly in developing fetuses, infants, and children. Although the US Food and Drug Administration (FDA) says that BPA is safe in low levels, one simple step you can take to play it safe, especially for the kids, is to favor BPA-free-labeled canned beans, tomatoes, and other products.

1. In a food processor, combine all the ingredients and process until smooth or with a few chunks remaining if you like. Taste and adjust the seasonings with more lime juice and/or salt if needed. If the dip is too thick, add a little more yogurt or some water, about 1 tablespoon at a time, until your desired consistency is reached.

2. Transfer to a bowl and serve immediately, garnished with the leftover cilantro if you like, or transfer to a container, cover, and refrigerate until you're ready to serve.

Variation:

Smoky Black Bean Dip: Omit the jalapeño and add 1/2 teaspoon smoked paprika or 1/2 to 1 teaspoon ground chipotle.

Zucchini Hummus

MAKES ABOUT 2 CUPS

Zucchini adds lightness to classic hummus and gets in a barely noticeable serving of veggies as a bonus. Tip: Don't peel your zucchini, as the majority of nutrients and fiber are in the skin.

+ 2 garlic cloves, peeled
+ 1 small zucchini, chopped
+ 1 (15-ounce) can no-salt-added chickpeas, rinsed and drained
+ 1/2 cup tahini (sesame paste)
+ 1/4 cup fresh lemon juice
+ 2 tablespoons extra-virgin olive oil
+ 1/2 to 1 teaspoon salt
+ 1/4 teaspoon freshly ground black pepper
+ *Garnishes:* extra-virgin olive oil, black olive slices, chopped parsley, paprika

Variations:

Roasted Red Pepper Hummus: Blend in 2 chopped roasted red peppers.

Herbed Hummus: After you've blended the hummus, add 1/2 cup chopped fresh dill, cilantro, mint, or parsley or a combination and pulse until well combined.

1. Combine all the ingredients in a food processor or blender and process until smooth, stopping to scrape the sides of the machine as needed, about 3 minutes.

2. Transfer to a bowl and serve immediately with the garnishes, or transfer to a container, cover, and refrigerate until you're ready to serve.

 Make Ahead: The dip will keep, covered and refrigerated, for up to 5 days, to have it handy for impromptu snacking throughout the week.

Hazards of Hummus and Other Dips

Packaged hummus can be a great time-saver, and it's easy to find all-natural brands in the supermarket. Look for ones that are low in sodium and made with olive oil and contain no added preservatives. Many other types of dip, on the other hand, tend to contain long, scary ingredients lists (the ones on the shelf tend to be worse than those in the refrigerated section), with unwanted add-ins such as MSG (monosodium glutamate) and artificial flavor, so be very careful when choosing; you may have better options in the natural foods section of the store, or go DIY (see the recipes on pages 41 to 60).

Pumpkin Seed Salsa

MAKES ABOUT 1½ CUPS

This simple version of a Maya Mexican staple is something new for most of us but destined to become a classic in your kitchen. Make sure to use hulled pumpkin seeds rather than those that come in the shell.

+ 1 cup raw unsalted hulled pumpkin seeds
+ 1 tablespoon extra-virgin olive oil
+ 2 medium plum tomatoes, chopped
+ 1 jalapeño chile, seeded and chopped
+ 1 garlic clove, pressed through a garlic press
+ 2 tablespoons fresh lime juice, or to taste
+ 1/2 bunch fresh cilantro, including stems, chopped
+ 1/2 teaspoon salt, or to taste

Continues ▶

Herbs: All in Good Taste

It might seem that herbs have only a tiny role to play in our overall health; we generally use them in such small amounts that it would make sense that their benefits are negligible. But just as adding a little seasoning can make a large impact on the flavor of a meal, scientists are finding that the cumulative use of different herbs offers a significant nutritional payload as well.

Herbs, including rosemary, thyme, basil, mint, and sage, all contain a vast array of powerful compounds, many of which have demonstrated antioxidant, anticarcinogenic, anti-inflammatory, and antiviral potential. They have also earned a reputation for aiding digestion and may even improve your general sense of well-being. If nothing else, herbs can help reduce our salt consumption and greatly enrich one of our favorite pastimes—eating!

1. Heat a medium skillet over medium heat. Add the pumpkin seeds and cook, stirring constantly, until lightly browned, about 5 minutes. Transfer to a food processor, cool for a few minutes, then add the oil and process until smooth, about 2 minutes, scraping the sides of the machine once or twice as needed.

2. Add the tomatoes, chile, garlic, lime juice, cilantro, and salt and process until smooth. Taste and adjust with more lime juice and/or salt if needed.

3. Transfer to a bowl and serve immediately, or transfer to a container, cover, and refrigerate until you're ready to serve.

Mint and Black Pepper Greek Yogurt Cheese or Dip

MAKES ABOUT 3/4 CUP CHEESE OR 1 CUP DIP

Did you know that Greek yogurt is just regular yogurt that's been strained to concentrate it (and thereby lessen its sugar content)? And if you strain it further, you have yogurt cheese to spread onto crackers or crudités for snacking. Add your herbs to Greek yogurt directly for the dip version, or strain your Greek yogurt first to make it cheese, or, even better, make a version of each!

+ 1 cup plain Greek yogurt
+ 1 tablespoon minced fresh mint
+ 1/4 teaspoon salt
+ 1/4 teaspoon coarsely cracked black pepper
+ Whole-grain crackers for yogurt cheese or vegetable sticks for dip

1. If you are making yogurt cheese, line a strainer with a paper towel or a piece of cheesecloth and set it atop a bowl tall enough to catch the liquid that drips out without touching the strainer. Place in the refrigerator overnight to strain.

2. Transfer the yogurt to a bowl (if you're making the dip, simply pour the yogurt into the bowl) and whisk in the mint, salt, and pepper. Taste, adjust the seasonings if needed, and serve with whole-grain crackers or vegetable sticks.

The New Pesto

MAKES ABOUT 1 CUP

Pesto makes anything it's added to, be it vegetables, fish, burgers, tofu, eggs, soup, or pizza, an instant gourmet meal. The New Pesto is inspired by your own creativity; it's about the classic basil and pine nut combo or switching up to include arugula, pumpkin seeds, walnuts, or whatever appeals to your palate. Have fun and experiment to come up with your own signature pesto!

If you're someone who thinks of pesto as an unhealthful food, consider the ingredients—nuts, Parmesan, lemon, garlic, and olive oil—and you'll see that it's actually pretty darn good for you. I'd much rather you dress up your pasta with pesto than go the standard alfredo route (unless, that is, it's the New Alfredo; see page 130 for the recipe).

+ 2 garlic cloves, peeled
+ 1/4 cup pine nuts, pumpkin seeds, walnuts, pecans, almonds, pistachios, or a combination, toasted (see page 209)
+ 2 cups packed fresh basil or a combination of basil and arugula, spinach, parsley, mint, or cilantro
+ 1 tablespoon fresh lemon or lime juice, or to taste
+ 6 tablespoons extra-virgin olive oil, or as needed
+ Salt and freshly ground black pepper
+ 1/4 cup grated Parmesan cheese

Garlic: The Brightest of Bulbs

Garlic is one of the oldest foods known to humankind and boasts a unique reputation among the healing traditions of the world. Garlic provides notable levels of vitamin C and B_6 as well as manganese and selenium, but the real excitement is generated around its sulfurous compounds, including allicin and alliin, which have been correlated with improved cardiovascular health, lowered blood pressure, and reduced risk of stroke. Its compounds demonstrate powerful antioxidant, anti-inflammatory, anticarcinogenic, and antiviral properties, and it has even been shown to help detoxify heavy metals and other toxins. If your friends can't stand the smell of garlic on your breath, then tell them why they need it and get them to eat some too!

1. Mince the garlic in a food processor by dropping it through the hole in the top while the processor is running. Add the nuts, herbs, lemon juice, and oil, season with salt and pepper, and process until smooth, stopping as needed to scrape down the sides of the bowl, about 1 minute.

2. Pulse in the cheese to combine. Taste and adjust the seasonings with salt, pepper, and/or lemon juice if needed. If your pesto is too thick, add a little water, and more water still for a thinner, sauce-like pesto.

3. To store your pesto, transfer it to a container, cover with a thin layer of oil, and refrigerate for up to 4 days, or freeze for up to 3 months.

Make Ahead: Having pesto on hand is a great tool for meal planning. To freeze pesto in single-serving portions, pour your pesto into ice cube trays and place in the freezer for 2 hours (if it goes much longer it can stick to the tray), then pop out the frozen pesto, transfer to freezer bags, and store in the freezer until ready to use.

Simply Tomato Salsa

No cooking repertoire is complete without a good tomato salsa recipe. Here we have two: salsa from scratch to take advantage of the bounty of the season, and salsa in a pinch, for when time is tight or a fresh, juicy tomato is but a distant warm-weather memory.

Tomato Salsa from Scratch

MAKES ABOUT 3 CUPS

+ 1½ pounds plum tomatoes (6 to 8), cored, cut in half, seeded, and cut into 1/4-inch pieces
+ 1/2 medium red onion, minced
+ 1 jalapeño chile, seeded and minced
+ 1 garlic clove, minced
+ 1/2 cup chopped fresh cilantro
+ 2 tablespoons fresh lime juice, or to taste
+ Salt to taste

In a large bowl, combine all the ingredients; if you have the time, let stand for 10 minutes to allow the flavors to come together before serving. The salsa will keep for up to 3 days in the refrigerator.

 Make Ahead: Make a batch or a double and use it freely as an Anytime Vegetable.

Tomato Salsa in a Pinch

MAKES ABOUT 3 CUPS

+ 3 cups low-sodium canned diced tomatoes, drained
+ 1/2 medium red onion, minced
+ 1 jalapeño chile, seeded and minced
+ 1 garlic clove, minced
+ 1/2 cup chopped fresh cilantro
+ 2 tablespoons fresh lime juice, or to taste
+ Salt to taste

In a food processor, pulse the tomatoes until roughly chopped, about 10 pulses. Pour into a fine-mesh strainer and drain for about 5 minutes, then transfer to a bowl and stir in the onion, jalapeño, garlic, cilantro, and lime juice. Season with salt. The salsa will keep for up to 5 days in the refrigerator.

Green Salsa

MAKES ABOUT 2 CUPS

The tomatillo, a tangy fruit hailing from Mexico, is an important part of the cuisine of that country and the star ingredient in this salsa. Typical green salsa has you roasting the tomatillos before blending; here we use raw tomatillos for a time-saving fresh-tasting green salsa. You'll find tomatillos in the produce aisle of the supermarket. They are housed in an inedible husk and covered in a slightly sticky coating; peel and rinse them well before using.

+ 1 garlic clove, peeled
+ 1 pound (about 12 medium) tomatillos, husked and rinsed
+ 1 to 2 jalapeño chiles, seeded and roughly chopped
+ 1/2 cup chopped fresh cilantro
+ 1/2 medium red onion, finely chopped
+ 1/4 to 1/2 teaspoon salt, to taste

1. Mince the garlic in a food processor by dropping it through the hole in the top while the processor is running.
2. Turn off the machine, add the tomatillos, chiles, and cilantro, then process to a chunky puree, adding a little water if the mixture is too thick.
3. Spoon into a bowl, stir in the onion and salt, and serve. The salsa will keep for up to 5 days in the refrigerator.

Puttanesca Salsa

SERVES 4

This take on the classic tomato, olive, and basil–based puttanesca sauce skips the cooking and goes light on the olives to keep the salt in check. To further cut down on salt, lightly rinse the olives before adding them. Serve the salsa with chicken or fish or anywhere you'd use standard tomato salsa.

+ 1 tablespoon extra-virgin olive oil
+ 1 tablespoon fresh lemon juice, or to taste
+ 1 teaspoon grated lemon zest
+ 1 garlic clove, pressed through a garlic press
+ 1/4 teaspoon crushed red pepper flakes
+ 1/4 teaspoon salt, or to taste
+ 1/4 cup pitted black olives, chopped
+ 1 pint cherry tomatoes, quartered
+ 1/2 cup chopped fresh basil

In a medium bowl, whisk together the oil, lemon juice, lemon zest, garlic, red pepper flakes, and salt. Add the olives, tomatoes, and basil, toss, and serve immediately.

Variation:

Cherry Tomato and Basil Salad: Omit the olives.

 Make Ahead: Make a batch to have handy to include in any meal or snack.

Corn and Red Onion Salsa

MAKES ABOUT 2 CUPS

There's nothing like freshly picked corn on the cob to celebrate summer. This light and colorful salsa is another way to further appreciate the anti-oxidant-rich, slightly sweet kernels. Serve aside chicken, fish, steak, or a burger, or straight from the bowl for snacking. Tip: Rub a lime wedge over grilled corn instead of slathering with butter for a fresh and lower-calorie finish to your cobs.

+ 2 ears corn, kernels cut from cobs
+ Pinch of baking soda
+ 1½ tablespoons fresh lime juice, or to taste
+ 2 teaspoons extra-virgin olive oil
+ 1/4 teaspoon salt, or to taste
+ 1 small to medium tomato, cored, seeded, and finely chopped
+ 1 small red onion, minced
+ 1/2 to 1 jalapeño chile, seeded and minced
+ 2 tablespoons chopped fresh cilantro

Make Ahead: Make a batch or a double and use it freely as an Any-time Vegetable.

Removing Kernels from a Cob

Cutting boards make for a messy corn kernel cutting station, with uncontained kernels making their way into unintended places. Instead, grab a large bowl and hold a shucked cob by the stem end with the tip of the ear resting at the bottom of the bowl. Cut the kernels from the cob using a sharp paring knife and they'll fall right into the bowl. A fun alternative is to use a Bundt pan: position the ear tip end down in the hole in the middle of the pan; shave off the kernels and they'll neatly drop into the bottom of the pan.

1. Bring a small pot of water to a boil over high heat. Add the corn, baking soda, and a pinch of salt and return to a boil. Remove from the heat and let stand for about 10 minutes. Drain and cool slightly.

2. In a medium bowl, whisk together the lime juice, oil, and salt. Add the corn, tomato, red onion, jalapeño, and cilantro and toss to combine. Let stand for about 15 minutes, then taste, adjust the seasonings with more salt and/or lime juice, and serve.

Variations:

Corn and Cucumber Salsa: Substitute 1 small peeled, seeded, and finely chopped cucumber for the tomato.

Corn and Pineapple Salsa: Substitute 1 cup finely chopped pineapple for the tomato.

Smoky Salsa: Add 1/4 teaspoon smoked paprika or 1/4 teaspoon chipotle powder and omit the jalapeño.

 Time-saver: Substitute 1½ cups frozen and defrosted corn kernels for the fresh corn.

Simply Tomato Sauce

MAKES ABOUT 3 CUPS

For all your tomato sauce needs—pasta, pizza, meat dishes, and more. Why not just open a jar instead? Because making your own means you have the tastiest sauce, and you get to be choosy with your ingredients: extra-virgin olive oil, organic tomatoes if your budget allows, salt and sugar levels at a healthy minimum, and no high-fructose corn syrup or artificial ingredients. For times when homemade isn't an option, look for bottles or cans that mirror the ingredients used here.

+ 2 teaspoons extra-virgin olive oil
+ 1 small yellow onion, chopped
+ 2 garlic cloves, chopped
+ 1 teaspoon dried oregano
+ 1 teaspoon Italian seasoning (optional)
+ 1/4 teaspoon red pepper flakes, or to taste
+ 2 teaspoons apple cider vinegar, or to taste
+ 1 (28-ounce) can no-salt-added crushed tomatoes
+ 3/4 teaspoon salt, or to taste
+ Up to 1 tablespoon pure maple syrup or honey, if needed

 Make Ahead: Make a batch or a double and use it freely as an Anytime Vegetable.

1. In a large saucepan, heat the oil over medium-high heat. Add the onion and sauté, stirring often, for about 7 minutes, until softened and browned. Reduce the heat to medium, add the garlic, and sauté for about 2 minutes, until softened. Add the oregano, Italian seasoning, if using, and red pepper flakes and cook for about 30 seconds, until aromatic, adding a tiny bit of water to the pan if the ingredients start to stick. Add the vinegar and stir to release all the delicious browned bits from the bottom of the pan.

2. Add the tomatoes and bring to a simmer, then cover, reduce the heat to low, and simmer for 10 to 30 minutes, according to how much time you have available (the flavors develop more as it cooks, but your sauce will still be delicious after 10 minutes). Taste and adjust the flavor with vinegar and/or salt if needed; if your tomato sauce is too tangy for your liking, add a little maple syrup.

Instant Guacamole

SERVES ABOUT 6 (MAKES ABOUT 2½ CUPS)

Instant Guacamole takes the guesswork out of everybody's favorite Mexican dip; if you have an extra few minutes, go for the Classic Guacamole. Both are best after resting for 15 to 30 minutes, once the flavors have taken some time to get acquainted.

And remember: guacamole is more than something to serve on a chip; it's equally at home with vegetable sticks (see the Anytime Vegetable list on page 101), alongside a fish, chicken, or other entrée, on a burger, atop nachos, or folded into scrambled eggs. Homemade guac is better than anything you'll find in a package, but if you don't have time to make your own, there are plenty of all-natural store-bought options to choose from.

+ 3 medium to large ripe avocados
+ 1/4 to 1/2 cup Simply Tomato Salsa (page 50) or jarred salsa
+ Fresh lime juice if needed

1. Cut the avocados in half, remove the pits, and scoop the flesh into a large bowl. Whisk them with a fork or mash with a potato masher to your desired texture, mixing in the salsa as you go, adding just enough to flavor the avocado without it becoming liquidy (if your salsa is on the liquidy side, scoop it out with a slotted spoon). Taste, add a little lime juice if the guacamole needs perking up, and serve immediately.

2. Cover with plastic wrap, placing it directly on the surface of the guacamole, and refrigerate until serving time.

Classic Guacamole

SERVES ABOUT 6 (MAKES ABOUT 2½ CUPS)

Step up your guac by using all fresh ingredients and it instantly becomes a classic!

- 3 medium to large ripe avocados
- 1/2 medium white or red onion, finely chopped
- 1 medium tomato, cored, seeded, and finely chopped
- 1/2 to 1 jalapeño chile, to taste
- 1/4 cup chopped fresh cilantro
- 1 tablespoon fresh lime juice, or to taste
- 1/4 teaspoon salt, or to taste

1. Cut the avocados in half, remove the pits, and scoop the flesh into a large bowl. Whisk them with a fork or mash with a potato masher to your desired texture, mixing in the remaining ingredients as you go.

2. Cover with plastic wrap, placing it directly on the surface of the guacamole, and refrigerate until serving time.

 Make Ahead: Make a batch to have handy to include in any meal or snack.

Six Simple Ways to Jazz up Your Guacamole

1. Bring on the Bacon Guacamole: *Add 2 strips of pork or turkey bacon, cooked until crisp and crumbled.*

2. Creamy Guacamole: *Mash the avocado until smooth (a whisk works well for this task), adding 2 tablespoons plain Greek yogurt as you go.*

3. Green on Green Guacamole: *Add Green Salsa (page 52) instead of tomato salsa.*

4. Corny Guacamole: *Add 1/2 cup fresh or frozen and thawed corn kernels.*

5. Sriracha Guacamole: *Use mild salsa and add a few squeezes of the Sriracha bottle.*

6. Smoky Guacamole: *Add 1/4 to 1/2 teaspoon chipotle powder, or smoked paprika for milder tastes.*

16 Sandwich Solutions

Feel free to mix and match and get creative here. Sandwich holder options include whole-grain bread or buns (if you're watching your carbs or calories, make it open-faced), whole-grain English muffins, whole-grain tortillas, or a collard leaf wrap—made by trimming the tough stem from a collard leaf, filling, and rolling as you would a tortilla. (This last option really cuts down on the carbs!)

1. **Smoky Black Bean Dip** *(page 43) sandwich with guacamole (page 59) or avocado slices*

2. **Zucchini Hummus** *(page 44) sandwich with salad greens*

3. **Pumpkin Seed Salsa** *(page 45) sandwich with No-Fry Falafel (page 125) or avocado slices*

4. **Mint and Black Pepper Greek Yogurt Cheese** *(page 125) sandwich with lettuce and tomato*

5. **Guacamole** *(page 59) sandwich with tomato and cheese*

6. **Pesto** *(page 48) tossed shredded chicken or crumbled tofu sandwich*

7. **"More Than Tuna" Tuna Salad** *(page 94) sandwich*

8. **Deconstructed Pesto Chicken Salad** *(page 157) sandwich with basil leaves*

9. **Orange, Fennel, and Rosemary Chicken Salad** *(page 156) sandwich with lettuce*

10. **Broccoli Chicken Salad** *(page 158) sandwich with mustard and tomato slices*

11. **Leftover Crispy Roasted Chicken** *(page 152) sandwich with hot sauce, shredded cheese, and shredded cabbage*

12. **No-Fry Falafel** *(page 125) sandwich with cucumbers and tomatoes*

13. **Instant Meatball** *(page 165) sandwich*

14. **Lime-Drenched Pork Salad** *(page 132) sandwich*

15. **Creamed Spinach** *(page 180) sandwich with shredded chicken or pork*

16. **Creamed Spinach** *(page 180) sandwich with avocado slices or guacamole (page 59)*

LABEL 411

What's in Your Bread Box?

When it comes to packaged bread, whole grain is the way to go. Whole grains are packed with fiber, minerals, and vitamins, so you want as much of that good stuff as possible! If the label doesn't boast 100 percent whole grain, you've only got a partial promise and there's a good chance a refined grain joins the list. Look for tricky wording to reveal white flour in disguise; examples include *wheat flour*, *unbleached wheat flour*, *enriched wheat flour*, *stone-ground wheat flour*, *100 percent wheat flour*—all have the all-important word *whole* absent.

Next, avoid hydrogenated oils, partially hydrogenated oils, and trans fats in favor of unrefined oils such as extra-virgin olive oil. Even sweeteners make their way into bread, often in the form of high-fructose corn syrup. Bread needs no added sweetener, but natural sweeteners such as honey are OK in small amounts. Many packaged breads contain a host of preservatives to give them their long shelf life and artificial colorings such as caramel coloring to give them a darker, misleadingly wholesome appearance. Avoid breads containing a color preceded by a number.

Not all bread is created equal, so check for serving sizes; oftentimes amounts are shrunk to give the appearance of fewer calories. While not for me, whole sprouted grain breads, often found in the freezer section, tend to be higher in nutrition, and the sprouting process makes the grains more digestible; these are worth a try for the adventurous. As with most foods, stick to breads with the shortest, healthy ingredients list!

Soups

For those of you new to from-scratch cooking, soup is an excellent place to test the waters. Start out with a good-quality stock and fresh veggies and it's hard to go wrong, as soup is a forgiving food, allowing you to adjust the seasonings, texture, consistency, and flavor until you're happy with your results. You can step up your soup by adding extra protein such as a leftover shredded chicken from last night's roast (page 159) or a handful of cooked chickpeas. Serve with a generous bowl of greens and you've made yourself a meal.

Just as chicken soup is Grandma's penicillin, by loading your soup with veggies and other heart-healthy ingredients, food will continue to be your medicine with every bowlful you sit down to.

Cool Cucumber Soup

SERVES 2 TO 3

Welcome relief from the heat on a steamy summer day, like salad in a glass. A great way to pack in the veggies!

+ 1 large cucumber, peeled and chopped
+ 1 cup plain yogurt
+ 1 cup cold low-sodium chicken stock (see the recipe on page 154 or use store-bought) or water
+ 1 small shallot, chopped
+ 1 garlic clove, chopped
+ 1½ tablespoons fresh lemon juice, or to taste
+ 1/4 teaspoon salt, or to taste
+ 1/4 teaspoon freshly ground black pepper
+ 2 tablespoons chopped fresh dill, plus more for serving if you like

1. In a blender or food processor, combine all the ingredients and blend until smooth. Taste and adjust the seasonings with more salt, pepper, and/or lemon juice if you like.

2. Spoon into bowls or glasses, top with dill, if using, and serve immediately, or pour into a container, cover, and refrigerate until cold before serving. The soup will keep refrigerated for up to 3 days.

LABEL 411

Stats on Stock and Broth

You may already know to look for low-sodium chicken stock (and if you don't, now you do!). Whether you're watching your sodium or not, choosing low-sodium means you're in charge of the amount of salt that goes into your soups, stews, and everything else. Avoid brands that contain caramel coloring to mimic the natural color of old-fashioned chicken stock. Stay clear of brands containing MSG; used to imitate the savory flavor of the chicken, MSG is unnecessary if your chicken stock is based on real chicken. Sometimes MSG will appear under aliases such as hydrolyzed vegetable protein, hydrolyzed plant protein, autolyzed plant protein, textured protein, or yeast extract, so be on alert when you come across an unrecognizable ingredient. (Side note: MSG has been used to induce obesity in laboratory animals, a good reason to stay clear of this additive!)

Add Veggies!
Add a handful of spinach leaves for extra green power.

Chilled Avocado and Herb Soup

SERVES 2 TO 4

I can't get enough of avocado—I bake an egg into it for breakfast (page 35), turn it into a spread in the form of guacamole (page 59), and blend it into this cooling yet satisfying summer soup. If you're wondering what else you can do with this creamy green fruit, turn to page 218 to turn your avocados into a dreamy chocolaty dessert!

+ 2½ cups low-sodium vegetable stock, chicken stock (see the recipe on page 154 or use store-bought), or water
+ 1 small avocado, peeled, pitted, and flesh scooped out
+ 1 small cucumber, peeled and chopped
+ 1 cup roughly chopped fresh cilantro (leaves and stems)
+ 1 cup roughly chopped fresh mint
+ 1 garlic clove, cut in half
+ 2 tablespoons fresh lime juice
+ Pinch of ground cayenne
+ 1½ teaspoons salt

1. Combine all the ingredients in a blender and blend until smooth, adding more stock or water if the soup is too thick. Taste and adjust the seasonings with more salt and/or lime juice if needed.

2. Serve immediately, or pour into a container, cover, and refrigerate until cold before serving. The soup will keep in the refrigerator for up to 2 days.

Avocado: A Good-Fat Fruit (Yes, It's a Fruit)

Avocados appear to have originated in Central America, being cultivated as early as 7,000 years ago. As we discussed in *The Doctor's Diet*, you shouldn't let their fat content scare you away—these are good, monounsaturated fats, and avocados are a nutritional powerhouse.

Avocados offer an invaluable spread of nutrients rarely found in a single food, with impressive levels of vitamins A, C, E, and B and minerals. They are full of fiber, and an avocado contains more than twice the amount of potassium than a banana. Eating avocado with your meals increases the absorption and assimilation of total nutrients, and several studies have found avocados can significantly lower bad cholesterol and raise good cholesterol. When you are watching your calorie intake, split your avocado with a friend!

Sweet Carrot Ginger Soup

SERVES 4 TO 6

You don't need cream to make a soup creamy! Here we add a small amount of rice to the soup as it cooks, and when it's blended the rice reveals its thickening powers, transforming your carrots into this dairy-free delicacy.

+ 2 teaspoons extra-virgin olive oil
+ 1 medium onion, chopped
+ 2 garlic cloves, chopped
+ 1 tablespoon chopped fresh ginger
+ 2 tablespoons raw brown rice

Continues ▶

- 1 teaspoon chili powder
- 1/4 teaspoon ground turmeric
- 1/8 to 1/4 teaspoon ground cayenne, to taste
- 1 pound carrots, sliced
- 6 cups low-sodium vegetable or chicken stock (see the recipe on page 154 or use store-bought) or water
- 1 teaspoon salt, or to taste
- 2 teaspoons grated orange zest, or to taste
- 1 tablespoon fresh lime juice, or to taste

---

1. Heat the oil in a large saucepan over medium heat. Add the onion and sauté until very soft, about 10 minutes. Add the garlic and ginger and cook for another 2 minutes, or until softened, adding a tiny bit of water to the pan if the mixture starts to stick. Add the rice, chili powder, turmeric, and cayenne and cook for 1 minute, stirring often, again adding a tiny bit of water to the pan if the mixture starts to stick.

2. Add the carrots, stock, and salt. Raise the heat to high and bring to a boil, then reduce the heat to low, cover, and simmer for 30 minutes. Stir in the orange zest.

3. Transfer the soup to a blender in batches if necessary and blend until smooth. Return the soup to the saucepan, adjust the seasonings, and stir in the lime juice. Taste and adjust the seasonings with salt, lime juice, and/or orange zest if necessary.

4. Spoon into bowls and serve.

Beet and Mushroom Barley Soup

SERVES 4 TO 6

I'll fess up—I've personally never developed a taste for beets, but I'm still trying because the health benefits are just so amazing (see the Beet Cancer! sidebar to learn about them). I think of this as a beginner beet recipe—light on the beets and heavy on the mushrooms and barley, just enough of the earthy red root to add a splash of color, not so much as to overtake.

+ 2 tablespoons extra-virgin olive oil
+ 1 medium onion, finely chopped
+ 2 medium carrots, finely chopped
+ 2 celery ribs, finely chopped
+ 3 garlic cloves, finely chopped
+ 1 pound white button mushrooms, thinly sliced
+ 3 tablespoons dry sherry or white wine (optional)
+ 6 cups low-sodium vegetable stock, chicken stock (see the recipe on page 154 or use store-bought), beef stock, or water
+ 2 medium beets, including stems if you've got them, peeled and finely chopped
+ 1/2 cup pearled barley
+ 1 teaspoon salt, or to taste
+ 1/2 teaspoon freshly ground black pepper
+ 2 tablespoons fresh lemon juice, or to taste
+ 1/2 cup chopped fresh dill, plus more for garnish
+ Plain Greek yogurt for topping (optional)

1. Heat the oil in a large saucepan over medium heat. Add the onion, carrots, and celery and cook until softened, about 5 minutes. Add the garlic and cook for about 2 minutes, until softened. Add the mushrooms and cook, stirring often, until the mushrooms are very soft, release their liquid, and the liquid evaporates, about 15 minutes. Add the sherry, if using, and cook until evaporated, about 2 minutes.

2. Add the stock, beets, barley, salt, and pepper and bring to a boil. Reduce the heat to low, cover, and cook, stirring occasionally, until the barley is softened, about 30 minutes. Stir in the lemon juice and season with more salt and pepper if needed. Stir in the fresh dill and beet greens, if using.

3. Spoon into bowls and serve, with more dill and yogurt as a garnish if you like.

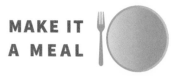

MAKE IT A MEAL Add shredded cooked beef to your finished soup.

Beet Cancer!

The medicinal qualities of beets have been respected since the days of ancient Greece. Beets contain a host of vitamins and minerals, particularly folate (commonly known as folic acid), potassium, and manganese, and beet leaves have been found to contain more iron than spinach.

But what's most exciting is that beets appear to earn most of their healing punch through the power of their phytonutrient pigments called betalains, which are powerful antioxidants. Beets have received a lot of attention as a complementary treatment in a wide range of cancers, and many cancer authorities put them at the top of their list of cancer-fighting foods. Beets also contain impressive levels of betaine, which is effective in metabolizing excess homocysteine in the blood, making it heart healthy, and it shows promise in the treatment of liver disease and depression as well as conditions of the blood, bones, and brain. Now you know why I'm trying so hard to learn how to enjoy eating them!

Red Lentil Soup

Unlike larger-size beans and chickpeas, red lentils cook quickly, in about a half hour, so there's no need to spend extra for the convenience of a can here. Millet adds a little texture and whole-grain goodness to this Moroccan-style lentil soup; if it's not available, it's fine to omit it.

+ 2 cups red lentils
+ 1/4 cup millet
+ 1 tablespoon extra-virgin olive oil
+ 1 large onion, finely chopped
+ 1 garlic clove, chopped
+ 2 tablespoons tomato paste
+ 1 tablespoon sweet paprika
+ 1/4 teaspoon cayenne pepper, or to taste
+ 9 cups low-sodium vegetable stock, chicken stock (see the recipe on page 154 or use store-bought), or water
+ 1 teaspoon salt, or to taste
+ 1 tablespoon finely chopped fresh mint
+ Plain Greek yogurt
+ Lemon wedges for serving

 Add Veggies! Add chopped carrots when you add the lentils, or throw in some spinach or other tender greens at the end of cooking.

Let's Eat Lentils

Most likely originating in central Asia, lentils have been cultivated for thousands of years, and they received some excellent PR in the Bible! Eating lentils and other legumes has been shown to reduce cholesterol, balance blood sugar, and lower the risk of heart disease, osteoporosis, and cancer.

One cup of lentils boasts exciting levels of B vitamins, including more than one's daily requirement for thiamin (B_1) and twice the daily requirement for folate. Lentils contain a ton of iron, magnesium, phosphorus, potassium, and zinc and even generous helpings of calcium and selenium. And don't forget the fiber and protein; that same cup of lentils contains a hefty wallop of protein (though it's lacking certain amino acids, which is why lentils and other legumes are often combined with grains in order to make a complete protein) and a substantial dose of fiber.

1. Place the lentils and millet in a fine strainer, rinse well, and drain.

2. Heat the oil in a large saucepan over medium heat. Add the onion and sauté until softened, about 5 minutes. Add the garlic and cook for 1 minute. Stir in the tomato paste, paprika, and cayenne and cook, stirring, for 1 minute.

3. Add the stock and stir to break up any stuck bits from the bottom of the pan. Add the lentils and millet, bring to a simmer, then reduce the heat to low, cover, and simmer for 30 minutes, or until the millet is cooked, the lentils have dissolved, and the mixture is thick, adding a little more stock or water if the mixture is overly thick. Stir in the salt.

4. Spoon into bowls and serve, topped with the mint and a dollop of yogurt, if using, with the lemon wedges on the side for squeezing.

"Not Just Chicken" Chicken Soup

SERVES 4

You need more than just chicken in your chicken soup! Veggies and whole grains take you beyond Grandma's penicillin to complete the "food as medicine" concept (and put a tasty meal on the table to boot).

For a reliable method of poaching chicken, simply follow the recipe through step 2, simmering the chicken in stock, draining, and shredding the meat. Poached chicken is perfect in recipes such as chicken salad (pages 156 to 158) and Quicksadillas (page 160).

+ 1 quart low-sodium chicken stock (see the recipe on page 154 or use store-bought)
+ 1 pound boneless skinless chicken breast
+ Salt
+ 2 carrots, sliced
+ 2 stalks celery, sliced
+ 1 bunch spinach, kale, or collard greens, stems removed, cut into thin strips or chopped
+ 1 cup cooked whole grain, such as brown rice, buckwheat, millet, or quinoa (pages 111 to 122; optional)
+ Handful of fresh herbs of choice, such as cilantro, parsley, dill, or mint
+ Freshly ground black pepper
+ Fresh lemon or lime juice

1. Pour the stock into a large saucepan and add the chicken. Season lightly with salt. Place over medium-high heat and bring to a boil,

Parsley: More Than Just a Garnish

Parsley is a respected herb that goes way back; physicians of ancient Greece extolled its numerous benefits, and Olympian athletes of the time were ceremoniously decorated with crowns of parsley. These days, parsley is more apt to appear as a token sprig in a restaurant meal, but there's reason to return it to its place of honor on the plate. Parsley is an exceptional source of vitamins C and A and folate, it's loaded with vitamin K, and it contains twice as much iron as spinach. It also delivers its very own suite of phytochemicals, which are steadily earning a reputation for potential therapeutic use (one such chemical, myristicin, has been shown to inhibit tumor formation and activate the body's detoxification systems).

There are many recipes in this book that pump up the flavor of parsley (the falafel recipe on page 125 uses a cup and a half of it, and the tabbouleh recipe above uses an entire bunch of it), making it more than just a garnish but a way of life!

skimming any foam that forms on top. Reduce the heat to low, cover, and simmer for about 10 minutes, until the chicken has just turned opaque throughout. (If you have an instant-read thermometer to use, it should read 165°F at the thickest part.)

2. Remove the chicken from the liquid and place on a plate to cool, then shred the chicken.

3. Return the chicken stock to a simmer, add the carrots and celery, and cook for about 5 minutes, until softened. Add the spinach and stir until wilted. Return the chicken to the pot, add the grain, if using, and stir to heat through. Stir in the herbs and season with salt, pepper, and lemon juice.

4. Spoon into bowls and serve.

Salads

If you're not a salad lover, here's my diagnosis: you've yet to learn how to make a tasty salad. I used to shy away from salads, but then as I started to vary my veggies, I developed a liking for them. But what turned my like to love was cheese: I don't need a creamy, calorie-heavy dressing to mask the flavors of my produce; all I need is a hint of real cheese, and just like that, I'm a salad lover. A little cheese goes a long way in dressing up a salad—include even the tiniest amount and a salad goes from ho-hum to yum, yum. My favorite is blue cheese, as its pungent flavor instantly kicks any salad up a few notches. Another way to guarantee a delicious salad: mash in an avocado for some good-fat, dressing-free creaminess, or just add sliced avocado chunks on top.

When you're really pressed for time, the supermarket offers any number of ways to jump-start your salad, from bags of chopped lettuce to prewashed mixed greens to coleslaw kits. Just be careful of salad kits that contain more than vegetables, as some slip in salty croutons, sugar-laden dressings, and other high-calorie ingredients.

Doctor's advice: don't pride yourself on "just eating a green salad for lunch." Chances are you'll add a boatload of unhealthy, processed dressing and you won't be satisfied without something substantial included in that salad. So don't be afraid to add a protein such as chickpeas or other beans, tofu, chicken, or fish. Adding protein, veggies, avocados, fruit, and, as I so often do, even a little cheese will turn your salad into a legit hunger-busting meal.

Everyday Green Salad
All Dressed Up

Not everybody has the same favorite vegetables, so you won't find a hard-and-fast recipe for making salad here. Instead, I'll share a list of mix-and-match choices arranged by taste and texture rather than write you a prescription for a set order of veggies (such prescriptions are often to blame for salad's bad rap). If you don't like one ingredient, go for another, taking care to get in plenty of greens.

A good dressing makes a great salad, and here I share four simple yet flavor-packed dressings that can be put together in minutes, almost as quick as it takes to pick out a bottle and bring it to the register. Feel free to add your own favorite dressings to your salad-making repertoire (stick to recipes using extra-virgin olive oil and minimal, if any, sweetener). And if you're truly pressed for time, there's nothing wrong with a quick toss with oil and vinegar—simply use a ratio of one part vinegar to two to three parts oil and you'll be good to go.

Grassy	arugula, asparagus, cabbage, chicory, endive, frisée, kale, romaine and other lettuce varieties, spinach, sprouts, watercress
Crunchy	beets, bell peppers, broccoli, carrots, cauliflower, celery, cucumber, green beans, jicama, onions, radishes, zucchini
Juicy/Creamy	avocado/guacamole, berries, tomatoes
Proteinaceous	beef, cheese, chicken, chickpeas/hummus, edamame (fresh soybeans), hard-boiled eggs, kidney beans, nuts, pork or turkey bacon, quinoa, shrimp, tofu, tuna, white beans
Herby	basil, chives, cilantro, dill, mint, oregano, parsley, scallions, thyme

1. Mix and match, heavy on the greens.
2. Lightly dress (see pages 80 to 83 for options), toss, and serve.

No Sweat Vinaigrette

- 2 tablespoons red or white wine vinegar, balsamic vinegar, or apple cider vinegar
- 1/4 teaspoon salt, or to taste
- Pinch of freshly ground black pepper
- 6 tablespoons extra-virgin olive oil

In a medium bowl, combine the vinegar, salt, and pepper, then whisk in the oil until emulsified.

Step It Up!

- Add 1 small garlic clove, pressed through a garlic press.
- Add 1 teaspoon minced shallot.
- Add 2 teaspoons minced fresh herbs.

Mustard Vinaigrette

MAKES ABOUT 3/4 CUP

+ 1/4 cup white wine vinegar or apple cider vinegar
+ 2 tablespoons Dijon-style mustard
+ 1/4 to 1/2 teaspoon salt, to taste
+ 1/4 teaspoon freshly ground black pepper
+ 1/2 cup extra-virgin olive oil

In a blender or food processor, combine the vinegar, mustard, salt, and pepper and blend until well combined. Slowly add the oil through the hole in the lid and blend until emulsified. Alternatively, combine all the ingredients except the oil in a medium bowl and whisk to dissolve the mustard, then whisk in the oil until emulsified.

Step It Up!

❖ Add 1 small shallot, minced, and/or 1 garlic clove, pressed through a garlic press.

Lemon Yogurt Dressing

MAKES ABOUT 3/4 CUP

+ 1/2 cup plain yogurt
+ 2 tablespoons extra-virgin olive oil
+ 2 tablespoons fresh lemon juice
+ 2 teaspoons grated lemon zest
+ 1 teaspoon Dijon-style mustard (optional)
+ 1 garlic clove, pressed through a garlic press
+ 1/4 to 1/2 teaspoon salt, to taste

In a blender or food processor, combine all the ingredients and blend until smooth. Alternatively, combine all the ingredients in a medium bowl and whisk to combine.

LABEL 411

Salad Dressing Surprises

Some folks eat salads just for the dressing, which isn't exactly the point, but a well-dressed salad can make the difference between an obligatory healthy dish and a truly tasty meal. There are countless kinds of dressings, and many of them are exceedingly unhealthy or at best have zero health value. The most flavorful dressings also tend to have the most fat, but this

Asian Sesame Dressing

MAKES ABOUT 1/2 CUP

+ 1 tablespoon rice vinegar or white wine vinegar
+ 2 tablespoons fresh lemon juice, or to taste
+ 2 teaspoons low-sodium soy sauce, or to taste
+ 2 teaspoons honey or pure maple syrup
+ 1 teaspoon toasted sesame oil
+ 1 teaspoon minced fresh ginger
+ 1 teaspoon minced garlic
+ 1/2 teaspoon salt, or to taste
+ 1/4 cup unrefined plain sesame oil or extra-virgin olive oil

In a blender or food processor, combine all the ingredients except the unrefined plain sesame oil and blend until smooth. Slowly add the oil through the hole in the lid and blend until emulsified. Alternatively, combine all the ingredients except the oil in a medium bowl and whisk to combine and dissolve the honey or maple syrup, then whisk in the oil until emulsified.

is not so much of a problem if those fats are good fats and they're used in moderation.

The most important thing to look for is the quality of the ingredients. Avoid hydrogenated oils and other highly refined vegetable oils, artificial colors and flavors, high-fructose corn syrup, and high levels of sugar and sodium in general. Look for unrefined oils like extra-virgin olive oil and short and simple ingredients you can pronounce!

Very Berry Arugula Salad

Tart, sweet, gorgeous to look at, and most important, a treat to eat. Try drizzling leftover dressing over fish.

Vinaigrette

+ 1/2 cup fresh raspberries
+ 2 tablespoons freshly squeezed orange juice or water
+ 1 tablespoon red wine vinegar or raspberry vinegar
+ 1 tablespoon honey or pure maple syrup (optional)
+ 1/4 teaspoon salt, or to taste
+ Freshly ground black pepper
+ 1/4 cup extra-virgin olive oil

Salad

+ 1 apple or pear, cored and sliced
+ 6 ounces (about 8 cups) arugula leaves
+ 1/2 cup toasted walnuts (see page 209)
+ 1/3 cup crumbled goat cheese (optional)
+ 1/3 cup fresh raspberries

1. To make the vinaigrette: Combine the raspberries, orange juice, vinegar, honey, if using, salt, and pepper to taste in a blender and blend until smooth. Stream in the oil in the hole through the top until emulsified.

2. To make the salad: In a large bowl, toss the apple slices with a little of the dressing. Add the arugula and more dressing (you will have leftover dressing) and toss to coat. Add the walnuts and goat cheese, if using, and toss lightly. Serve immediately topped with the raspberries.

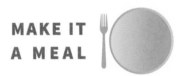

MAKE IT A MEAL

Add leftover shredded chicken and serve over a bed of quinoa or other whole grain (pages 111 to 122).

Mighty Green Salad

Get past your lettuce! Once you're really into an eat-your-greens groove, salad becomes an adventure in variety, as in this lettuce-less hearty green salad.

+ 1 bunch collard greens (about 1 pound), thick stems removed and leaves cut into thin strips
+ 2 small heads bok choy
+ 1/4 to 1/2 teaspoon salt
+ 2 large carrots, coarsely grated
+ 2 scallions, light and green parts, thinly sliced
+ 2 tablespoons toasted sesame seeds
+ Asian Sesame Dressing (page 83)

1. In a large bowl, combine the collard greens and bok choy. Add the salt and massage the greens with your hands for about 2 minutes, until they start to wilt. Add enough dressing to coat (you will have leftover dressing) and massage the dressing into the salad to further wilt the greens. Add the carrots, scallions, and sesame seeds and toss.

2. You can serve the salad now, or refrigerate it for a couple of hours, tossing occasionally, for 1 to 3 hours or overnight.

Cruciferous Crusaders

Cruciferous vegetables belong to the brassicas, a family of potent veggies that includes broccoli, cabbage, cauliflower, kale, bok choy, collards, mustard greens, and Brussels sprouts among others. They're equipped with variable amounts of vitamins and minerals, but much of the fuss about brassicas concerns their phytochemical payload. Phytochemicals are the biologically active compounds found in plants, and there are hundreds of studies examining the potential health benefits of these compounds, pointing to powerful anticarcinogenic and detoxification properties. It is our detoxification system that grabs hold of unwelcome guests such as pollution and food additives and swiftly escorts them off the premises, so the more you favor crucifers, the greater your chances are of keeping clean inside.

Throughout this book we explore a number of creative ways of working with cruciferous veggies. Some of these crucifers may be at the top of your list, while others may be a bit closer to the bottom—no problem; just choose the ones you like and put them on the menu!

 Make Ahead: Because we're using sturdy greens, you can make the salad a day ahead of serving without fear of it becoming soggy.

Cucumber Caprese Salad

SERVES 4 TO 6

The classic caprese—an Italian tomato, mozzarella, and basil salad—just got crunchier with the addition of cucumber, and lettuce leaves complete the salad experience. For big-time basil lovers, skip the vinaigrette and toss with pesto (page 48) thinned with a little olive oil or water.

+ 4 ounces fresh mozzarella cheese, cut into 1/2-inch pieces (about 1/2 cup)
+ 1 pint cherry tomatoes, cut in half
+ 1 medium cucumber, peeled, seeded, and cut into 1/2-inch pieces
+ 1 cup fresh basil leaves, chopped
+ 1 romaine heart, quartered lengthwise and cut into 1/2-inch pieces
+ About 2 tablespoons No Sweat Vinaigrette (page 80)

1. In a large bowl, combine the cheese, tomatoes, cucumber, basil, and romaine heart. Add the dressing and gently toss to coat.
2. Divide among plates and serve.

Step It Up!
For the crispest caprese, toss your halved tomatoes with 1/4 teaspoon salt, place them in a colander set over the sink, and let drain for 15 minutes to 1 hour, stirring occasionally, before composing your salad.

Why Buy Local?

There is growing evidence to indicate that fresh produce is higher in nutrition than produce that has been in storage and shipping for days and weeks. Many fruits (tomatoes, bananas, avocados, and peaches, for example) are picked unripe so that they can be trucked thousands of miles without rotting. However, it is in that final ripening phase that many nutrients reach their maximum potency. For instance, tomatoes that are picked before ripening have been found to have less vitamin C and lycopene than vine-ripened tomatoes. Other studies have shown a clear decrease of nutrients over time once produce has been harvested. A tomato that was harvested ripe by a local farmer yesterday is likely to have a lot more going for it than an unripe tomato that was harvested weeks ago on the other side of the country.

But you don't really need a study to know all that—just trust your taste buds and you'll know what's best!

The New Cobb Salad

SERVES 4

Here's a trimmed-down version of the classic and a meal in a bowl. For a crispy finish, top with Chickpea Crunch (page 89).

+ 8 ounces boneless skinless chicken breast, poached according to the instructions on page 75 and chopped
+ 1 cup cherry tomatoes, cut in half
+ 1 head romaine lettuce, chopped

Continues ▶

- About 1/4 cup No Sweat Vinaigrette (page 80) or Mustard Vinaigrette (page 81)
- 2 large hard-boiled eggs, chopped
- 2 slices cooked pork or turkey bacon, crumbled
- 1 ripe avocado, cut in half, pitted, and chopped
- 1 ounce blue cheese, crumbled (about 1/4 cup)

1. Combine the chicken, tomatoes, and lettuce in a large bowl and toss with dressing to coat.

2. Divide into bowls, top each with hard-boiled egg, bacon, avocado, and blue cheese, and serve.

Step It Up!
Toss the chicken, tomatoes, and lettuce with dressing separately and serve traditional Cobb style by lining a salad platter with horizontal rows of each ingredient.

 Time-saver: If roasted chicken is on the dinner menu tonight, use leftover chicken breast to make the salad tomorrow.

Summer Squash Ribbon Salad

SERVES 4

This warm-weather salad takes crisp-tender shavings of colorful summer squash, perks them up with lemon, adds Parmesan for some salty deliciousness, and finishes with a nice little sunflower seed crunch. See page 214 to learn more about the benefits of these seeds.

+ 1 pound summer squash (yellow or a mix of yellow and green)
+ 2 tablespoons extra-virgin olive oil
+ 1 tablespoon fresh lemon juice
+ Salt and freshly ground black pepper
+ 1 cup baby arugula
+ 1/4 cup shaved Parmesan (shaved with a vegetable peeler)
+ 1 tablespoon toasted sunflower seeds or pumpkin seeds

1. Trim the ends from the squash and, using a vegetable peeler, thinly slice the squash lengthwise into strips and place them in a large bowl.

2. Add the oil and lemon juice, season with salt and pepper to taste, and toss. Let stand for a few minutes, then toss with the arugula. Scatter the Parmesan on top and sprinkle with the sunflower or pumpkin seeds. Serve immediately.

Variation:

Asparagus Ribbon Salad: Substitute asparagus for some or all of the summer squash (trim the tough woody ends before slicing).

 Make Ahead: The squash can be sliced into ribbons and refrigerated a few hours before assembling.

Sweet and Tangy Kale Salad

SERVES 4

Not too long ago, kale was the stuff of health food fanatics; now kale chips are all the rage (see my recipe on page 206) and kale is a star salad ingredient. All that's needed is a quick massage with dressing to make it tender like lettuce. If you're not a fan of kale (I won't judge you!), try substituting an equal amount of thinly sliced cabbage for a tangy take on coleslaw.

+ 1 large bunch Tuscan kale (the flat-leaf type), stems removed
+ 2 tablespoons extra-virgin olive oil
+ 1 to 2 tablespoons fresh lemon juice, to taste
+ 1 small garlic clove, pressed through a garlic press
+ 1/4 teaspoon salt
+ 1/4 teaspoon freshly ground black pepper
+ 1 large carrot, finely grated
+ 1/2 cup toasted walnut halves (see page 209)
+ 1/4 cup raisins
+ 3 tablespoons grated Parmesan cheese

1. Stack the kale leaves on a cutting board and roll them up like a cigar, then thinly slice them crosswise.

2. In a large bowl, whisk together the oil, lemon juice, garlic, salt, and pepper. Add the kale and use your hands to massage the dressing into the leaves until they soften and wilt. Toss the carrot with the kale to coat it with the dressing. Add the walnuts, raisins, and cheese and toss well. Taste and adjust the seasonings with more salt, pepper, and/or lemon juice if needed.

Step It Up!

❖ After massaging the kale, let sit for 10 minutes to 1 hour to soften it and bring the flavors together, or refrigerate overnight.

❖ Soak the raisins in warm water for 30 minutes to plump them before adding to the salad (you can do this while the kale is marinating).

"More Than Tuna" Tuna Salad

SERVES 2

A real tuna salad's got some real salad in it—loaded not just with tuna but veggies too! Take the salad concept one step further and serve over lettuce leaves, or fix yourself a good old tuna salad sandwich, open-faced or closed depending on how closely you're watching your carbs today. Tip: If one veggie isn't to your liking, simply double up on another.

+ 1 (5-ounce) can chunk white tuna in water or olive oil
+ 1 medium bell pepper, cored, seeded, and finely chopped
+ 1 small carrot, finely chopped
+ 1 small celery stalk, finely chopped
+ 1 scallion, finely chopped
+ 3 to 4 tablespoons olive oil mayonnaise
+ 2 teaspoons Dijon-style mustard
+ 1 teaspoon fresh lemon juice, or to taste
+ 1/4 teaspoon salt, or to taste
+ 1/4 teaspoon freshly ground black pepper
+ Lettuce leaves or 2 to 4 slices whole-grain bread

1. Place the tuna in a large bowl. Add the bell pepper, carrot, celery, scallion, mayonnaise, mustard, lemon juice, salt, and pepper and stir with a fork to combine, breaking up any large chunks of tuna as you

A Buyer's Guide to Fish

Fish continues to be a pivotal source of food for people around the world, providing exceptional nutrition and health benefits. But because of the pollution in our waters, a certain measure of consumer awareness is called for.

Varying levels of mercury in particular have been found in many fish, so it's best to be careful if your intake is more than 12 ounces a week. Certain fish, mostly the larger, predatory species (like swordfish, tilefish, and king mackerel), should be avoided because as they eat smaller fish, the level of mercury increases in concentration. It's a good idea to check advisories about the safety of fish caught in local lakes, rivers, and coastal areas. Pregnant women, nursing mothers, and young children should exercise particular caution around eating the wrong kind of fish.

Generally speaking, wild-caught fish tends to be more nutritious and has a better balance of essential fatty acids than farmed fish. (Not to mention that farmed salmon is often injected with pink dye to mimic the carotenoid pigments of wild salmon!) The Monterrey Bay Aquarium maintains a website called Seafood Watch (seafoodwatch.org) with the latest science-based recommendations on safe and responsible seafood consumption. They have also released a printable pocket guide and an app you can have handy so you won't feel like a fish out of water when you get to the store. For consumption advisories about fish in your local waters, check out the US Environmental Protection Agency's "Advisories Where You Live" feature at fishadvisoryonline.epa.gov.

go. Taste and adjust the consistency and seasonings, adding more mayonnaise, lemon juice, or salt as needed.

2. Serve over lettuce as a salad or on crusty bread to make sandwiches.

Veggie-Full Sides

Adding a dedicated side to your meal is an excellent way to elevate your cooking—that is, if you have the time. But don't worry, as always, you have options. For example, you can make the Green Beans with Toasted Coconut (page 104) to serve alongside the Chicken Curry (page 101). But if you're in a hurry to make your curry (who says a cookbook can't rhyme?!), simply cook the green beans into the chicken. Once you learn a little multitasking, you'll be able to make both without any extra time spent in the kitchen. And don't forget your Anytime Vegetables; see the list on page 101 for the simplest side ideas.

Roasted Vegetables 101

YIELD VARIES

Clear out those pots and pans you've got stored in the oven and make way for the veggies! Roasting vegetables is nothing short of an act of transformation, resulting in a side that's crispy on the outside, tender inside. Roasting caramelizes the natural sugars in the vegetables, bringing out their sweetness, and flavors are concentrated to make those veggies more delicious. All you need is a working oven, a baking sheet or two, olive oil, and seasonings and you're ready to roast.

Refer to the chart on page 100 for roasting time ranges, and use 450°F as your base temperature.

+ About 2 pounds vegetables
+ 1 to 2 tablespoons extra-virgin olive oil
+ Salt and freshly ground black pepper to taste
+ Sprinkle of herbs of choice, such as oregano, rosemary, sage, thyme, or parsley

1. Preheat the oven to 450°F and line a baking sheet or two with parchment paper or aluminum foil.

2. Trim or peel the vegetables as needed. Cut the vegetables into even-size pieces. Place the vegetables in a large bowl. Add the oil and toss well to fully coat the vegetables in the oil. Season with salt and pepper and add herbs, if using, and toss well again.

Tips for Roasting Vegetables

❖ Mix and match vegetables with similar roasting times.

❖ Toss your vegetables with the oil and seasonings in a bowl (rather than directly on the pan) to evenly coat them.

❖ Be generous: vegetables will shrink while roasting as they lose their liquid. Take that into consideration as you plan your portions.

❖ Don't overcrowd the pan; leave a little space between the pieces so they roast rather than steam.

❖ Cut the vegetables into uniform pieces so they cook evenly.

❖ Check and turn your vegetables halfway through roasting time.

❖ If the vegetables are browning too quickly, lower the oven temperature.

3. Arrange the vegetables on the baking sheet in a single layer, leaving space between them so they don't overlap. Place in the oven and roast according to the chart, turning them halfway through roasting, until the vegetables are tender on the inside and golden brown and crisp on the outside.

Asparagus	tough ends snapped off	10 to 15 minutes
Bell peppers	1-inch-wide strips	30 to 35 minutes
Broccoli	2-inch florets (stems peeled and chopped)	10 to 15 minutes
Brussels sprouts	outer leaves and stem trimmed, cut in half through the stem end	15 to 20 minutes
Carrots	1-inch pieces	35 to 40 minutes
Cauliflower	1½-inch florets	20 to 30 minutes
Eggplant	½-inch pieces	20 to 30 minutes
Green beans	ends trimmed	20 to 30 minutes
Mushrooms (button)	stems trimmed	20 to 30 minutes
Onions (large)	peeled and cut into 10 to 12 wedges	20 to 30 minutes
Parsnips	peeled and cut into thin strips	15 to 20 minutes
Potatoes (fingerling, purple, red-skinned)	2-inch pieces	40 minutes
Sweet potatoes	2-inch pieces	40 minutes
Tomatoes (plum)	halved lengthwise, cored and seeded, cut side up	20 to 30 minutes
Winter squash (acorn, butternut, delicata, kabocha)	2-inch pieces	45 minutes
Zucchini	1-inch slices	15 to 20 minutes

Anytime Vegetables: A Simple Side-Dish Solution

Enjoy ample amounts of any of these vegetables with breakfast, lunch, and dinner and anytime in between.

Alfalfa sprouts

Artichoke hearts

Artichokes

Asparagus

Bamboo shoots

Bean sprouts

Beets

Beet greens

Bell peppers (red, orange, yellow, green)

Bok choy

Broccoli

Broccoli sprouts

Brussels sprouts

Cabbage (green or red)

Carrots

Cauliflower

Celery

Chiles

Cilantro

Collard greens

Cucumbers

Eggplant

Endive

Fennel

Garlic

Grape leaves

Green beans

Jicama

Kale

Kohlrabi

Leeks

Lettuce (any kind)

Mesclun (mixed greens)

Mushrooms

Mustard greens

Nori and other sea vegetables (try seaweed snacks)

Okra

Onions

Parsley

Peas

Pumpkin

Radishes

Rhubarb

Rutabaga

Salsa (pages 50 to 54)

Scallions

Snow peas

Spinach

Squash (acorn, butternut, delicata, Hubbard, spaghetti, yellow summer)

Swiss chard

Tomatillos

Tomatoes

Tomato sauce (page 56)

Turnips

Turnip greens

Vegetable juice

Watercress

Yellow wax beans

Zucchini

Leafy Greens Made Easy

SERVES 4

Doctor's orders: eat your greens at every opportunity! Here are three simple methods—steaming, blanching, and sautéing—to do so deliciously.

+ 1 pound tender or hearty greens (see box)
+ 1 tablespoon extra-virgin olive oil, or to taste
+ 1 to 2 garlic cloves (if sautéing)
+ Fresh lemon or lime juice
+ Salt and freshly ground black pepper
+ Herbs or spices (optional)

Remove the stems from hearty greens and tear the greens into bite-size pieces, then choose your method: steaming, blanching, or sautéing.

To steam your greens:

1. Set a steamer insert or a colander into a saucepan filled with about an inch of water, just enough to come below the bottom of the steamer without touching. Place over medium heat and bring to a simmer. Place the greens in the steamer insert, cover, reduce the heat to low, and cook until wilted, about 2 minutes for tender greens, about 5 minutes for hearty greens.

2. To shortcut steam your greens, put them in a microwave-safe bowl. Don't add water; the water remaining on the leaves after washing will be enough to steam them (if they come prewashed, add a splash of water). Cover with microwave-safe plastic wrap, leaving one corner open to vent, and steam as above.

To blanch your greens:

Bring a large saucepan of water to a boil. Add the greens and cook for 30 seconds to 1 minute for tender greens or about 3 minutes for hearty greens. Drain, cool slightly, then squeeze out excess water.

To serve steamed or blanched greens:

Toss with olive oil, add a squeeze of lemon juice, and season with salt and pepper to taste and herbs if you like.

To sauté your greens:

1. Heat the oil in a large skillet over medium heat. Add the garlic and sauté for 1 minute, or until golden.

2. Start adding the greens in batches (using tongs works best) until the skillet is starting to fill up but not overflowing. Once the greens start to cook down, add more in batches until all of the greens are in and wilted. If the pan starts to get dry, add a splash of water to partially steam the vegetables (adding water rather than more oil keeps the calories down). Add lemon juice to taste and season with salt and pepper to taste and herbs if you like.

Tender greens	Hearty greens
bok choy	collard greens
dandelion greens	kale
mustard greens	
spinach	
Swiss chard	
turnip greens	

Green Beans with Toasted Coconut

SERVES 6

Simple use of flavorings and spices—in this case coconut and lemon juice—makes a veggie dish feel like more than a mere veggie but a newfound friend that you'll call upon again and again. It pairs with Chicken Curry (page 148), or if you don't have the time to make both a main and a side, simply add cut green beans to your curry during the last 5 to 10 minutes of cooking time.

+ 12 ounces green beans, cut into 1-inch pieces (see Time-saver below for options)
+ 2 teaspoons extra-virgin olive oil
+ 2 tablespoons unsweetened dried coconut
+ 1 tablespoon fresh lemon juice, or to taste
+ Pinch to 1/4 teaspoon ground cayenne, or to taste
+ 1/4 teaspoon salt

1. Bring a large pot of water to a boil. Add the green beans and cook until just cooked through and bright green, about 3 minutes. Drain and set aside.

2. Heat the oil in a large skillet over medium-high heat. Add the coconut and cook, stirring, for 10 to 20 seconds, until it starts to color (watch the pan carefully, as coconut can burn easily).

3. Turn off the heat and stir in the green beans (or heat them through if you've made them in advance). Add the lemon juice, cayenne, and salt and stir to coat the beans. Taste, adjust the seasonings, and serve.

 Time-saver: Buy precut green beans in a microwave-ready bag and microwave them instead of blanching them in water, or use frozen green beans.

Brussels Sprouts Confetti

SERVES 4

You don't need to eat Brussels sprouts to be healthy, but then again, there's no reason not to! When they're very thinly sliced and lightly dressed, Brussels sprouts are fresh tasting, like a mini version of cole-slaw, and add a festive feeling to your food. Toss with any light dressing or keep your confetti unembellished; use as a bed for Perfectly Seared Steak (page 173) or serve alongside a fish or other main dish. The recipe scales up easily for all you Brussels sprouts lovers out there.

+ 8 raw Brussels sprouts
+ About 1 tablespoon No Sweat Vinaigrette (page 80), Mustard Vinaigrette (page 81), or another dressing (optional)

1. Cut the stem end off of the Brussels sprouts, remove the outer leaves if necessary, and very thinly slice to create "confetti."
2. Place the Brussels sprouts in a large bowl. Add the dressing, if using, and toss to coat.

Garlicky Butternut Squash Mash

SERVES 4

Who's got the time to peel and chop squash and sweet potatoes? Going for frozen is a real time-saver here, and combining this duo of orange-fleshed favorites makes for a not too dense, not too light, just right mash.

+ 2 teaspoons extra-virgin olive oil
+ 1 teaspoon finely chopped fresh ginger
+ 2 garlic cloves, finely chopped
+ 1 (10-ounce) package frozen sweet potato chunks, defrosted
+ 5 tablespoons milk
+ 1 (10-ounce) package frozen butternut squash chunks, defrosted
+ 1/2 teaspoon salt, or to taste
+ Pinch of ground nutmeg (optional)
+ 2 teaspoons fresh lemon juice, or to taste

Variation:

All-Squash Mash: Use 2 (10-ounce) packages butternut squash and omit the sweet potatoes; decrease the cooking time to 10 minutes.

1. Heat the oil in a large saucepan over medium heat. Add the ginger and garlic and cook, stirring, for 2 to 3 minutes, until softened. Add the sweet potatoes and milk, bring to a simmer, then reduce the heat to low, cover, and simmer for about 10 minutes, until almost completely softened. Add the squash and salt, cover, and cook for another 5 minutes, or until both the sweet potatoes and squash are completely softened.

2. Transfer to a food processor, add the nutmeg, if using, and the lemon juice and process until smooth. Taste and adjust, then serve.

Cauliflower Steak

SERVES 4 TO 5

A steak that's easy to love for vegetarians and meat eaters alike!

+ Extra-virgin olive oil cooking spray
+ 1 medium head cauliflower
+ Salt and freshly ground black pepper

1. Preheat the oven to 450°F and spray a baking sheet with cooking spray.

2. Remove the leaves and carefully trim the base of the cauliflower core but don't remove it. Stand the cauliflower upright and cut it length-wise into 3/4-inch slices. The center slices should remain more or less intact, but the outer slices may crumble. That's OK; they'll still be delicious after they're roasted.

3. Put the slices and any crumbles on the baking sheet, spray with cook-ing spray, and season with salt and pepper to taste. Roast until the tops are browned in places and the stems are easily pierced with a fork, about 30 minutes, turning halfway through. (If there are any crumbles on the sheet, they most likely will cook more quickly; check when you turn the steaks and remove the crumbles from the baking sheet if they're starting to brown.) Serve with a knife and fork.

10 Ways to Spice Up Your Cauliflower Steak

1. Sprinkle with lemon zest and lots of cracked black pepper.

2. Drizzle with toasted sesame oil instead of the cooking spray and sprinkle the finished steaks with toasted sesame seeds and minced scallions.

3. Sprinkle 1 tablespoon minced garlic over the steaks before roasting.

4. Substitute smoked paprika for the black pepper when roasting.

5. Add 1/4 cup shredded Parmesan cheese during the last 5 minutes of roasting.

6. Finish with lemon juice and minced parsley.

7. Top with Simply Tomato Salsa (page 50) or Green Salsa (page 52).

8. Drizzle with salad dressing (pages 80 to 83).

9. Top with pesto (page 48).

10. Serve with steak sauce.

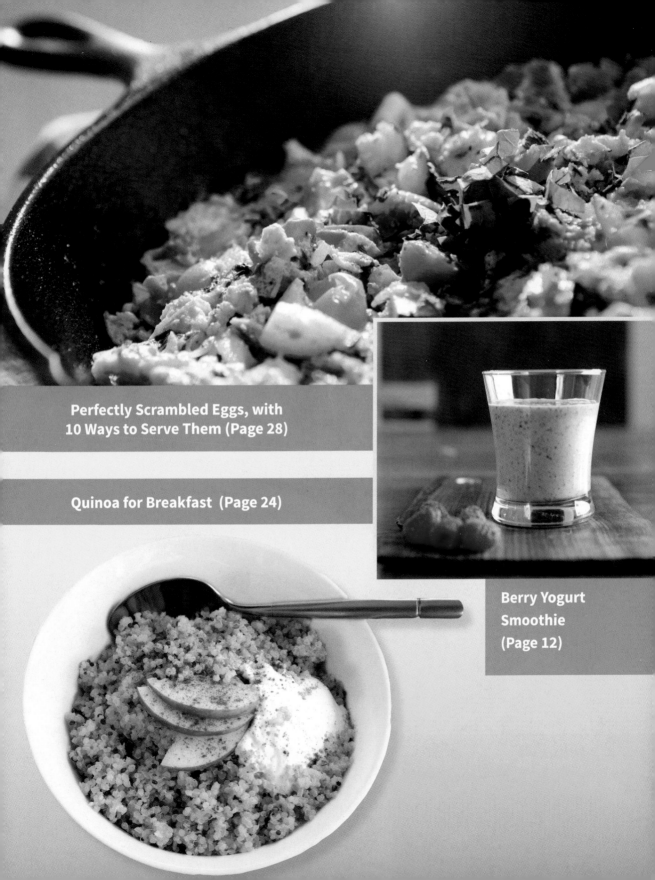

Perfectly Scrambled Eggs, with 10 Ways to Serve Them (Page 28)

Quinoa for Breakfast (Page 24)

Berry Yogurt Smoothie (Page 12)

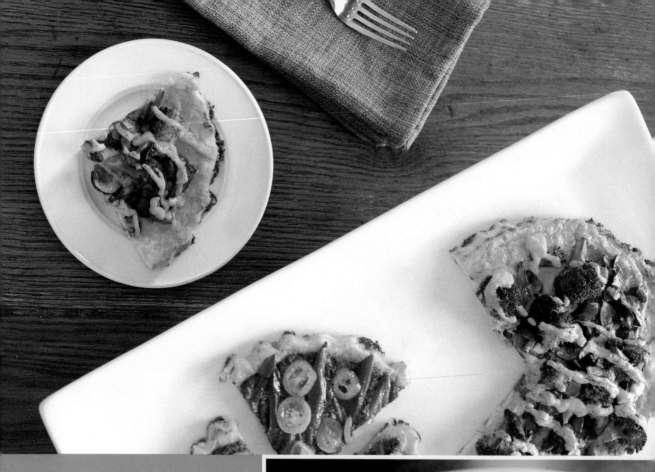

**Cauliflower Crust Pizza
(Page 182)**

**Classic Burger (Page 189)
with Zucchini Fries (Page 191)**

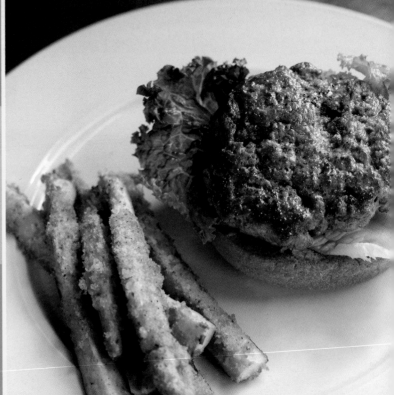

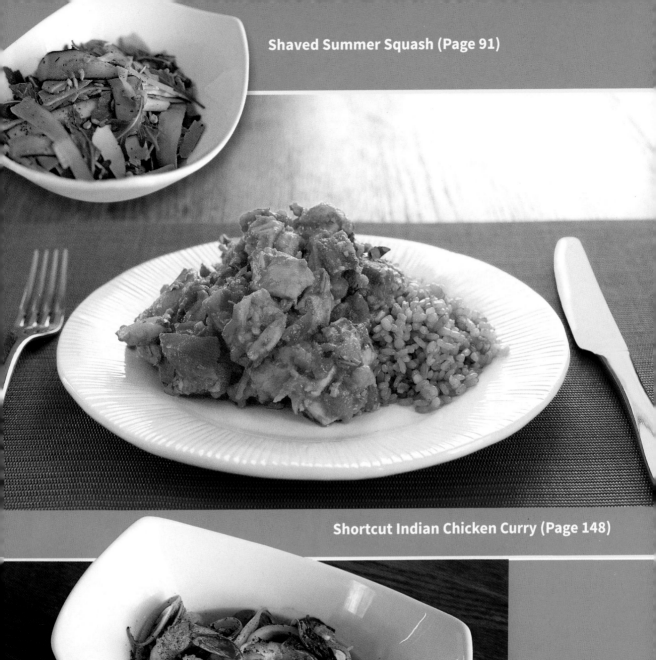

Shaved Summer Squash (Page 91)

Shortcut Indian Chicken Curry (Page 148)

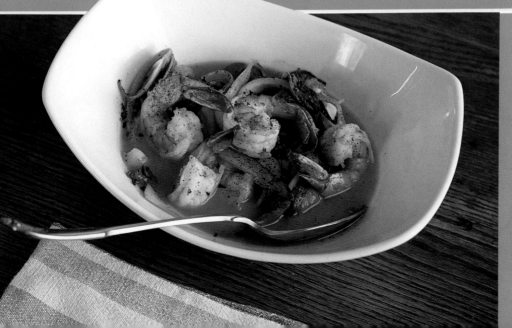

Poached Shrimp (Page 145)

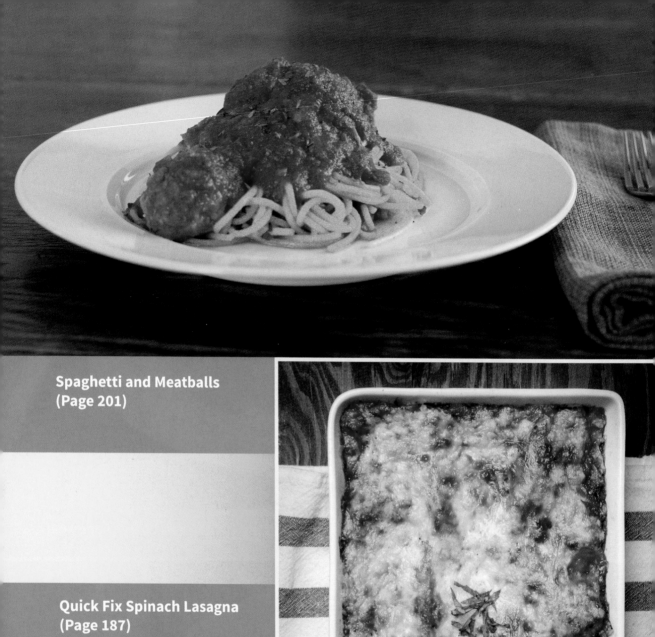

**Spaghetti and Meatballs
(Page 201)**

**Quick Fix Spinach Lasagna
(Page 187)**

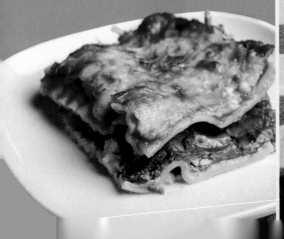

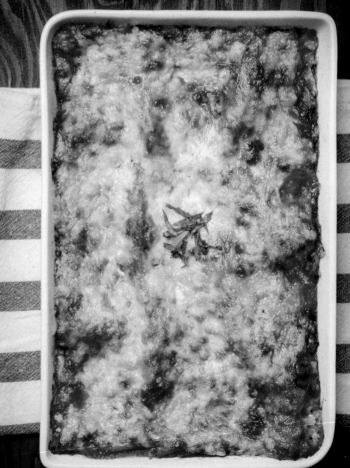

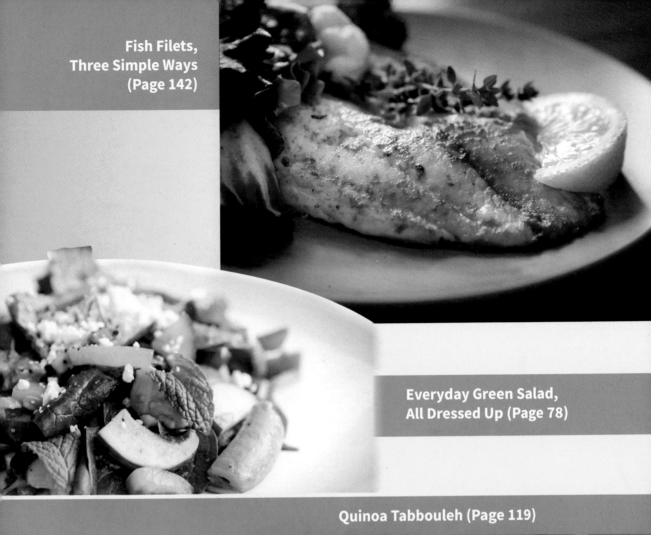

Fish Filets, Three Simple Ways (Page 142)

Everyday Green Salad, All Dressed Up (Page 78)

Quinoa Tabbouleh (Page 119)

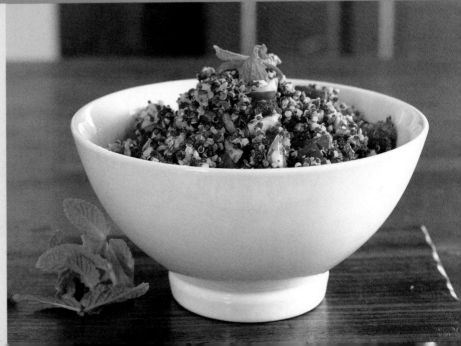

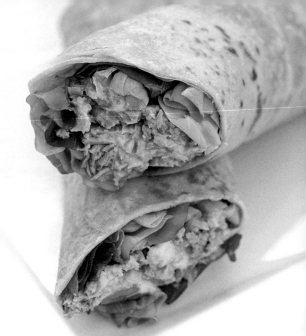

**Super-Quick Tuna Melt
(Page 159)**

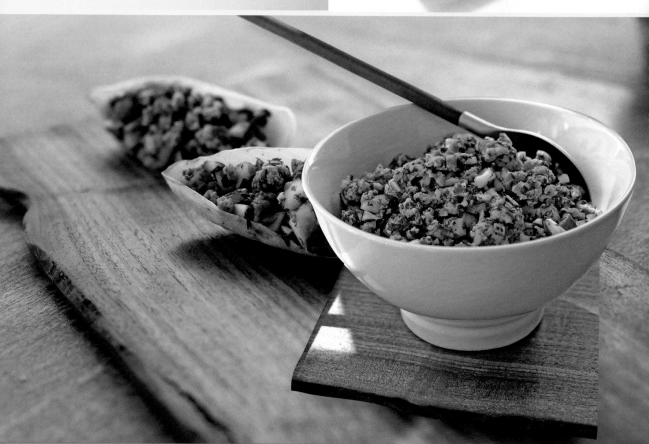

Limey Thai Ground Pork Salad (Page 132)

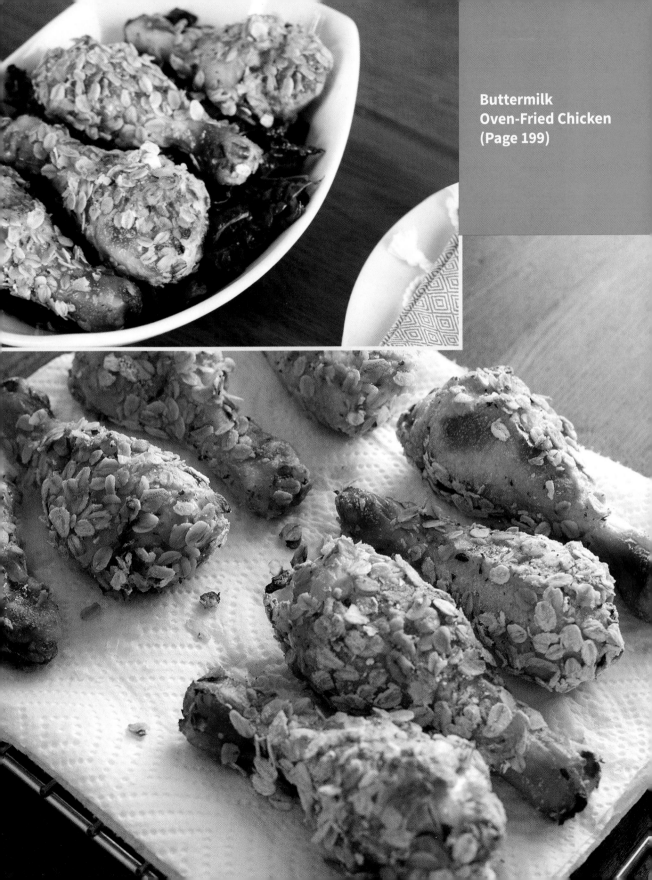

**Buttermilk
Oven-Fried Chicken
(Page 199)**

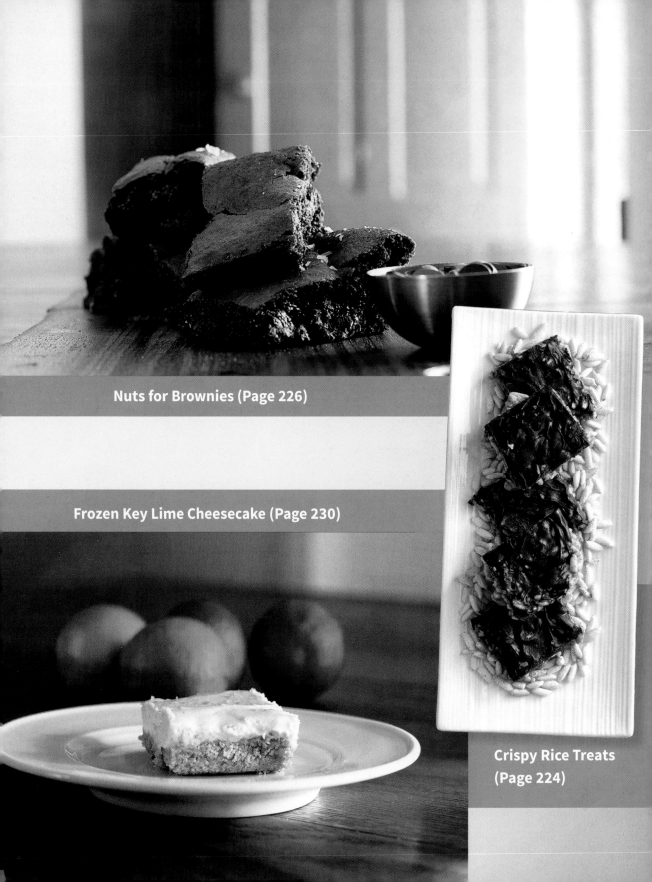

Nuts for Brownies (Page 226)

Frozen Key Lime Cheesecake (Page 230)

Crispy Rice Treats (Page 224)

Nudels

SERVES 2

Here's a fun and healthful alternative to wheat-based pasta and a great way to make use of a bumper crop of zucchini. All that's required is a box grater, but if you get really into zucchini noodle making, you might look into purchasing a spiral vegetable cutter, a nifty little hand-cranked gadget that will turn any number of vegetables, from carrots to winter squash to sweet potatoes, into noodles. This gadget is sold in kitchen stores and online. Serve your nudels in any recipe that calls for traditional pasta; they're perfect tossed with pesto.

+ 2 large zucchinis

1. With the large holes of a box grater facing down lengthwise over the zucchini, pass the grater over the zucchini, pressing firmly in long strokes to create strands of noodles. When you approach the seeds, turn the zucchini and shred the other side. (Toss the remaining seedy part into a soup or use it in your hummus; page 44.)

2. To serve your nudels in the nude, place them in a colander for about 15 minutes to release some of their moisture, then wrap them in paper towels and lightly squeeze to absorb the moisture before dressing and serving. If nude is not for you, briefly boil, sauté, or microwave your nudels and serve.

Spaghetti Squash: Another Nudel Option

Preheat the oven to 400°F. Make steam vents in a spaghetti squash by pricking it deeply with a paring knife. Place on a baking sheet and bake for about 1 hour, until softened (press it to check). Cut the squash in half lengthwise and scrape out and discard the seeds and fibrous part in the middle. Hold one half with a kitchen towel to protect your hand and use a spoon or fork to scrape the flesh out of the peel and into a bowl, keeping the strands as intact as you can. Top with a simple drizzle of olive oil and salt and pepper or any sauce you like, or use in place of traditional noodles in any recipe.

Whole-Grain Sides

It's simple: when you go for a grain, make it a whole grain. Whole grains are filled with protein, fiber, and vitamins and minerals, unlike their stripped-of-nutrition refined counterparts. The fiber in whole grains may help lower your risk of heart disease, diabetes, and certain cancers, and is guaranteed to leave you feeling satisfied while eating less. Low-carb diets are all the rage these days, but I take a middle ground: avoid the refined carbs and make whole grains a core component of an overall healthy balanced diet. And if you're gluten-free, skip the wheat and stick to gluten-free whole grains, avoiding products containing substitute ingredients like gums and starches that don't contain nutritional value.

This chapter includes simple instructions for preparing five whole grains—brown rice, buckwheat, millet, quinoa, and whole-wheat couscous, with a stepped-up variation of each for when you've got a little extra time. Grains freeze well; package them in single-serving portions and reheat as needed.

Basic Brown Rice

MAKES ABOUT 3 CUPS

It may be basic, but brown rice isn't always a cinch to make. Many people complain of rice that's overcooked and mushy or undercooked and crunchy. Boiling your rice pasta-style avoids both extremes for a perfect pot every time. And there's nothing wrong with using either ready-to-boil or microwave brown rice if that's what best fits in with your kitchen routine. (I fully admit to doing so!)

+ 1 cup brown rice (long-grain, short-grain, or basmati)
+ 1/4 teaspoon salt, or to taste

1. Rinse the rice well in a strainer under cold running water.

2. Bring a large pot of water to a boil over high heat and add a little salt. Add the rice, stir, then reduce the heat to medium and boil for 30 minutes, stirring a couple of times.

3. Pour the rice into the strainer and drain well, shaking the strainer a few times. Return the rice to the pot (do not turn on the heat), cover, and set aside to steam and absorb excess moisture for 10 minutes. Uncover, fluff the rice with a fork, season with salt, and serve. If you're not using your rice right away, spread on a large plate to cool, then transfer to a container and refrigerate or freeze.

Brown Rice with Asparagus, Peas, and Toasted Almonds

SERVES 6 AS A SIDE

+ 1 recipe Basic Brown Rice (see page 112)
+ 1/2 bunch asparagus, woody ends trimmed off, stalks chopped
+ 1/2 cup frozen and defrosted or fresh peas
+ Handful of toasted slivered almonds

Make the rice as directed above, adding the asparagus during the last 3 minutes of cooking. When you return the rice to the pan (after draining it and), add the peas, then fluff and serve topped with the almonds.

MAKE IT A MEAL 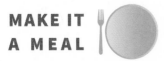 Serve topped with a poached egg.

Beans and Rice in a Pinch

This quick fix is my go-to when I'm shooting in LA and the days are long with little time for dinner. I'll often make enough to last for three nights; sometimes I'll swap in another whole grain such as quinoa, and when I've had a slow activity day, I'll go light on the grain or simply omit it.

Combine ready-to-boil brown rice, microwavable brown rice, or leftover cooked brown rice with no-salt-added canned black beans. Add salsa, guacamole, shredded cheddar cheese, and hot sauce to taste, mix, and serve.

Basic Buckwheat

MAKES ABOUT 3½ CUPS

Buckwheat actually has no relation to wheat and is technically classified as a fruit seed in the rhubarb family. Buckwheat is a great source of quality protein and is a nutrition treasure trove; notably it contains a phytochemical called rutin, which is known for its antioxidant, anti-inflammatory, and anticarcinogenic effects. It has also been shown to balance blood sugar and reduce the risk of stroke. In most nutrient categories, buckwheat surpasses wheat, and because it is gluten-free it is more digestible for people who are sensitive to wheat.

When it's toasted, buckwheat is referred to as kasha; the two can be used interchangeably.

+ 1 large egg white
+ 1 cup buckwheat groats
+ 1/4 teaspoon salt, or to taste

1. Beat the egg white in a medium bowl and add the buckwheat; toss to coat.

2. Heat a large saucepan over medium heat, add the buckwheat, and cook, stirring constantly, until the grains are dry and no longer clumping together, about 3 minutes. Add 1½ cups water and the salt, cover, increase the heat to high, and bring to a boil. Lower the heat and simmer until the water is absorbed and the buckwheat is tender, about 10 minutes.

3. Remove from the heat and let stand, covered, for 5 minutes, then fluff with a fork. If you're making your buckwheat in advance, spread on a large plate to cool, then transfer to a container and refrigerate or freeze.

Variation:

Vegan Buckwheat: Omit the egg and toast the buckwheat in the pan with 2 teaspoons extra-virgin olive oil, stirring often, until fragrant, about 3 minutes, then proceed with the recipe.

Protein-Packed Buckwheat

SERVES 6 AS A SIDE

+ 1 recipe Basic Buckwheat (see above)
+ 1/2 cup cooked lentils (half of a 15-ounce can, rinsed and drained)
+ 2 teaspoons apple cider vinegar
+ 1/4 cup chopped fresh parsley, dill, or mint

Prepare the buckwheat as directed above. Just after you turn off the heat, add the lentils, cover, and let stand for 5 minutes, then fluff with a fork, mixing the lentils into the buckwheat. Stir in the vinegar and parsley and serve.

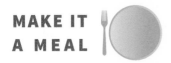

MAKE IT A MEAL Serve with a salad (pages 77 to 94).

Basic Millet

MAKES ABOUT 4 CUPS

Millet's not just for birds; I'm sure you'll agree if you give it a try, either as a simple side or stepped up with mangos, yogurt, and seasonings to The Sweet Side of Millet. Reasons to enjoy your millet: it has a rich amino acid profile and is high in magnesium, phosphorus, B vitamins, and iron, and it easily cooks to a light, fluffy pilaf texture with little effort. (To give it more of a mashed potato texture, bump up the water to 3 cups and increase the cooking time to about 40 minutes.)

If you're not using your millet right away, spread it on a large plate or baking sheet to cool (this prevents it from clumping), then transfer to a container and refrigerate or freeze.

+ 1 cup millet
+ 1/4 teaspoon salt, or to taste

1. Rinse the millet well in a strainer under cold running water.

2. In a large saucepan, combine the millet, 2½ cups water, and the salt, cover, bring to a boil over medium-high heat, then reduce the heat to low and simmer until the millet is tender and the liquid is absorbed, 20 to 25 minutes.

3. Let stand, covered, for 5 to 10 minutes before fluffing with a fork and serving.

Step It Up!
For a nutty flavor and aroma, toast the millet in the pan over medium-high heat, stirring constantly, until fragrant, 3 to 4 minutes, before adding the water.

The Sweet Side of Millet

SERVES 6 AS A SIDE

- 1/4 cup plain yogurt
- 2 tablespoons fresh lime juice, or to taste
- 2 teaspoons chili powder
- 3/4 teaspoon salt
- 1 recipe Basic Millet (see page 116), hot or at room temperature
- 1 red bell pepper, cored, seeded, and finely chopped
- 1 jalapeño chile, seeds removed, minced
- 1 medium ripe but firm mango, peeled, pitted, and cut into 1/2-inch pieces
- Leaves from 1/2 bunch fresh cilantro, roughly chopped

In a large bowl, whisk together the yogurt, lime juice, chili powder, and salt. Add the millet, red pepper, jalapeño, mango, and cilantro and stir to combine well. Taste and adjust the seasonings with salt and/or lime juice if needed.

MAKE IT A MEAL 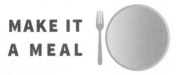 Add chickpeas and serve over a bed of lettuce or shredded cabbage.

Basic Quinoa

Quinoa is a modern superfood with age-old roots that's enjoyed for its nutty flavor, crunchy yet light texture, and high protein content. Read more about the quinoa backstory on page 171.

+ 1 cup quinoa
+ 1/4 teaspoon salt, or to taste

1. Rinse the quinoa well in a strainer under cold running water.
2. In a large saucepan, combine the quinoa, 1½ cups water, and the salt, cover, bring to a boil over medium-high heat, then reduce the heat to low and simmer until the quinoa is tender and the liquid is absorbed, 15 to 20 minutes.
3. Let stand, covered, for 5 to 10 minutes before fluffing with a fork and serving.

Quinoa Tabbouleh

SERVES 6 AS A SIDE

+ 1 recipe Basic Quinoa (see page 118), at room temperature
+ 2 medium ripe tomatoes, chopped
+ 1/2 medium red onion, finely chopped
+ Finely grated zest and juice of 1 large lemon, plus more lemon juice if needed
+ 1 garlic clove, pressed through a garlic press
+ Leaves from 1 large bunch fresh flat-leaf parsley, finely chopped
+ Handful of fresh mint leaves, finely chopped

Step It Up!
After combining the quinoa with the onion, lemon zest and juice, and garlic, let the mixture sit for 30 minutes so the flavors can combine to their fullest.

Place the quinoa in a large bowl. Add the tomatoes along with their juices, then add the onion, lemon zest and juice, and garlic and stir well. Add the parsley and mint and stir to combine. Serve at room temperature, or cover and refrigerate for up to 3 days and serve cold.

Variations:
* Use 3 chopped scallions in place of the onion.
* Substitute arugula for half of the parsley.
* Add 1 seeded and diced cucumber to the salad.

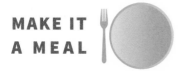

MAKE IT A MEAL Add cooked shredded chicken or cubed firm tofu.

Basic Whole-Wheat Couscous

MAKES 2½ CUPS

Couscous goes from dry to cooked in five minutes and pairs with just about everything, making it a staple for weeknight dinners.

Tip: Never boil couscous, even if the directions on the package tell you to do so (it will come out soggy); follow the directions below for reliably al dente couscous.

+ 1 cup instant whole-wheat couscous
+ 1/4 teaspoon salt, or to taste

In a small saucepan, bring 1 cup plus 1 tablespoon water to a boil, turn off the heat, then stir in the salt and couscous. Let stand, covered, for 5 minutes, then fluff with a fork.

Zesty Couscous with Summer Squash

SERVES 6 AS A SIDE

- 1 tablespoon extra-virgin olive oil
- 1 medium yellow onion, chopped
- 1 medium yellow squash, cut into thin half-moons
- 1 medium zucchini, cut into thin half-moons
- 1½ teaspoons grated lemon zest
- 1 recipe Basic Whole-Wheat Couscous (see page 120)
- 1/2 cup toasted pine nuts
- 1/3 cup raisins, soaked
- 1/2 teaspoon freshly ground black pepper
- 1 tablespoon fresh lemon juice, or to taste
- Salt

1. In a medium saucepan, heat the oil over medium heat. Add the onion and sauté until softened, about 5 minutes. Add the yellow squash and zucchini and sauté for another 3 minutes, or until slightly softened. Remove from the heat, stir in the lemon zest, and set aside.

Continues ▶

Step It Up!
Soak the raisins in warm water for 30 minutes to plump them before adding to the couscous.

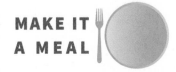 **MAKE IT A MEAL** Add shredded chicken and serve over a bed of spinach.

Zucchini: Endlessly Adaptable

You'll notice that zucchini (a type of summer squash) makes several appearances in the book. Because of its mild flavor and soft but pliable texture, it's endlessly adaptable and takes on the flavor of whatever it's cooked, tossed, or blended with, be it sautéed with a grain as we've done here, ground into hummus (page 44), shaved into ribbons (page 91), turned into noodles (page 109), or baked into fries (page 191), making it easy to love for even the staunchest of veggie skeptics out there!

2. Transfer the couscous to a large bowl and stir in the onion-squash mixture, pine nuts, raisins, pepper, and lemon juice. Taste and add more salt to taste and/or lemon juice if needed.

Mains

Popular cooking shows aside, you don't have to be a master chef to be the star of your home kitchen! If you've got time to cook just one full meal today, make it a main; better yet, make it a double so you'll have leftovers for tomorrow. There's no shame in using supermarket shortcuts to get your dinner to the table—bags of shredded cabbage and carrots, cut green beans, chopped peppers, asparagus, and so on—if your budget allows; you'll still be saving lots by not eating out.

These mains bypass borders, with globally inspired dishes that even a novice can tackle, and there's something for everyone—from vegans and vegetarians to meat eaters and the gluten-free among us. Recipes to live for!

No-Fry Falafel

MAKES ABOUT 30 FALAFELS

Granted this isn't likely to be your everyday go-to, but if you're feeling adventurous, give it a whirl! The method is pretty simple—no more than mix, roll, and bake, for a healthy homemade falafel (restaurant falafel is typically fried) that will serve you for several meals. I like my falafel veggie-heavy, so I pack it with parsley. To make your falafel gluten-free, substitute chickpea flour (see page 39) for the whole-wheat flour.

Falafel

+ 2 cups dried chickpeas
+ Extra-virgin olive oil cooking spray
+ 1 small onion, chopped
+ 3 garlic cloves, chopped
+ 1½ cups chopped fresh parsley leaves or a mix of parsley and cilantro
+ 3 tablespoons whole-wheat flour, plus more if needed
+ 2 tablespoons water
+ 1/2 teaspoon baking soda
+ 2 teaspoons ground cumin
+ 1 teaspoon ground coriander
+ 1/2 teaspoon sweet paprika
+ 1/4 teaspoon ground cayenne, or to taste
+ 1 teaspoon salt, or to taste
+ 1/2 teaspoon freshly ground black pepper

Continues ▶

 Time-saver: Swap the tahini sauce with Greek yogurt.

Make Ahead: The falafel will keep for up to 5 days in the refrigerator or in the freezer for 2 to 3 months (pop into the toaster oven to reheat).

Tahini Sauce

- ✚ 3/4 cup tahini (sesame butter)
- ✚ 3/4 cup water, or as needed
- ✚ 2 teaspoons honey (optional)
- ✚ 1½ tablespoons fresh lemon juice, or to taste
- ✚ 1½ teaspoons freshly grated lemon zest
- ✚ 3/4 teaspoon sweet or smoked paprika
- ✚ 1/4 teaspoon salt, or to taste

1. To make the falafel: Put the chickpeas in a large bowl and add water to cover by about 4 inches. Cover with a dish towel and soak for about 24 hours, checking a couple of times that they remain covered with water and adding more if needed. They will double in size. Drain and rinse the chickpeas.

2. Preheat the oven to 425°F and spray two baking sheets with cooking spray.

3. Place the chickpeas, onion, garlic, parsley, flour, water, baking soda, cumin, coriander, paprika, cayenne, salt, and pepper in a food processor. Pulse the mixture until it is just short of pureed, with a coarse and grainy texture to it, stopping the machine to scrape down the sides

Time-saver: Use 2 (15-ounce) cans chickpeas, drained and rinsed, for the dried chickpeas. Skip the soaking and go straight to mixing up the batter. The batter will be moist, so you probably won't need to add water.

Introducing the Falafel Waffle

Gently stuff a whole-grain pita with 2 or 3 falafels and spray both sides of the pita with extra-virgin olive oil cooking spray. Place in a pre-heated waffle iron, close, and bake for 3 to 5 minutes, until the falafel merges with the pita to create a falafel waffle. There's just enough room in your pita to fit your falafel (the waffle iron won't close if the pita is overly full), so the sauces and add-ins go on top of your finished waffle. This is the most fun you'll ever have with falafel, and feel free to try it with any number of other sandwich fillings!

once or twice and adding a little water if needed to get the machine going. Check the mixture: it should stick together when you pinch it a bit with your fingers. If it's too runny, add a little more flour; if it's too thick, add a little water. Transfer to a large bowl.

4. Roll the chickpea mixture into approximately 1½-inch balls (use a spring-release cookie scoop if you've got one), flatten them with your hands into patties, and place them on the prepared baking sheets. Spray the tops with cooking spray. Place in the oven and bake on one side for about 10 minutes, until golden, then flip the falafels and bake on the second side until the outside is crusty and the inside is still soft, 10 to 15 minutes more.

5. While the falafel is baking, make the tahini sauce: In a medium bowl, whisk together all the ingredients until smooth. Taste and adjust the seasonings if necessary and add more water if the sauce is too thick.

Serving Suggestions

❖ Whole-wheat pita bread or wraps or lettuce leaves
❖ Hummus (homemade, page 44, or store-bought)
❖ Lettuce, tomatoes, and cucumber

Summer Sesame Noodles

SERVES 4

Peanut butter, garlic, ginger, and other simple seasonings combine to make a silky sauce for this veggie-heavy take on a Chinese-American restaurant staple. Soba, a Japanese-style noodle based on buckwheat (those who are gluten-free can look for 100 percent buckwheat soba), can be found in natural food stores and some supermarkets; if unavailable, feel free to use whole-wheat spaghetti. Add a handful or two or Chickpea Crunch (page 205) for a little extra texture and protein if you like.

Dressing

+ 1/3 cup smooth all-natural no-sugar-added peanut butter, tahini (sesame paste), or a combination
+ 3 tablespoons low-sodium soy sauce
+ 1/3 cup warm water or low-sodium vegetable stock, or as needed
+ 2 teaspoons minced peeled fresh ginger
+ 2 garlic cloves, pressed through a garlic press
+ 3 tablespoons rice vinegar
+ 2 teaspoons toasted sesame oil
+ 1 tablespoon honey or maple syrup
+ 1/2 teaspoon dried red pepper flakes

Noodles

- 8 ounces cooked and cooled soba noodles or whole-wheat spaghetti
- 1 cup cubed firm or extra-firm tofu
- 1 medium cucumber, peeled, cut in half, seeds scooped out, and thinly sliced
- 2 scallions, thinly sliced
- 1 red or orange bell pepper, cored, seeded, and thinly sliced
- 1 cup fresh mint leaves, chopped
- 3 tablespoons toasted sesame seeds (optional)

---

1. Make the dressing: Combine all the dressing ingredients in a blender and blend until smooth; add more water if the dressing is too thick. Transfer to a large bowl.

2. Add the noodles, tofu, cucumber, scallions, bell pepper, and mint and toss to coat well. Garnish with the sesame seeds, if using, and serve.

Add Veggies!
Massage 1/2 bunch kale, stemmed and very thinly sliced, into a little of the dressing before adding the noodles and remaining ingredients.

The New Alfredo

SERVES 4 TO 6

This creamy pasta dish is gluten- and dairy-free comfort food, with anti-inflammatory and antioxidant protection provided by the "cream" from the cruciferous vegetable cauliflower. Top with crumbled pork or turkey bacon and you'll put it over the top.

- 3 tablespoons extra-virgin olive oil, plus more if needed
- 6 cloves garlic, sliced lengthwise
- 2 medium heads cauliflower, cut into florets
- 1 teaspoon salt, or to taste
- 8 ounces whole-wheat or brown rice linguine
- 2 teaspoons dried oregano
- 1/2 teaspoon red pepper flakes, or to taste
- 1 (15-ounce) can cannellini beans, drained and rinsed
- 2 teaspoons apple cider vinegar, or to taste
- Freshly grated Parmesan cheese, for serving (optional)

1. Combine 2 tablespoons of the oil and the garlic in a large skillet, place over medium heat, and cook, stirring, for about 3 minutes, until the garlic begins to turn golden.

2. Raise the heat to medium and add the cauliflower, salt, and 1/4 cup water. Cover the skillet and cook, stirring occasionally, for about 20 minutes, until the cauliflower has softened, breaking up larger pieces with a potato masher as the cauliflower cooks and coarsely mashing it as it finishes cooking.

3. Meanwhile, bring a large pot of water to a boil, salt it, add the pasta, and cook until al dente. Drain.

4. Add the oregano and red pepper flakes to the cauliflower and cook for 2 minutes; add the drained pasta, beans, and vinegar and cook for another 2 minutes or so to warm the pasta and beans through, adding a little more water if the sauce is too thick. Stir in the remaining 1 tablespoon of olive oil. Taste and add more salt and vinegar if needed.

5. Spoon into bowls and serve, sprinkled with cheese if you like.

Lime-Drenched Pork Salad Ⓢ

This take on a classic Thai/Laotian dish called larb *makes liberal use of lime and fish sauce to give it that signature Southeast Asian taste; with generous amounts of fresh cilantro, mint, and red onion, you've got yourself a dinner salad. Chicken, turkey, lamb, or another meat can be substituted for the pork.*

Serve over brown rice or another grain as a main, or try it spooned onto crisp lettuce or Napa cabbage leaves as a side. Leftovers make a tasty sandwich filling.

If you are watching your sodium, you might scale back on the fish sauce, as it is rather salty; luckily you only need a little to get a lot of flavor. You can find fish sauce in Asian markets or the Asian food section of your grocery store.

+ 1 pound ground lean pork
+ 3 tablespoons fresh lime juice, or to taste
+ 2 tablespoons fish sauce, or to taste
+ 1/2 medium red onion, chopped
+ 3/4 cup chopped fresh mint
+ 3/4 cup chopped fresh cilantro or basil
+ Whole grain of your choice (pages 111 to 122) or crisp lettuce leaves for serving

1. Add the pork to a large skillet, place over medium-high heat, and cook until it is no longer pink and is browned in places, about 10 minutes, breaking up the meat with a wooden spoon as you cook it. Transfer to a serving bowl to cool until warm or room temperature, stirring it a few times.

2. In a small bowl, combine the lime juice and fish sauce; pour the mixture over the pork and stir to coat. Add the red onion. Taste and add additional lime juice and/or fish sauce if needed. Stir in the mint and cilantro and serve over a whole grain or atop lettuce leaves.

 Make Ahead: Squeeze the limes, combine the juice with the fish sauce, and chop the herbs ahead of time; later all that's needed is to cook the pork, toss, and serve.

Festive Fish Tacos

MAKES 8 TACOS

When you make your tacos from scratch, you know you'll be getting the best-quality ingredients possible, and your figure will thank you for steaming the fish instead of frying it like they do at the corner taco joint. For your taco base, pass on the white flour tortillas in favor of 100 percent corn tortillas or another additive-free whole-grain tortilla (read your labels; see opposite page), or go virtually carb-less by piling your fish and toppings onto crisp lettuce or Napa cabbage leaves or tender turnip slices.

Fish

+ 1½ pounds skinless cod or other firm white fish fillet, sliced 1/4-inch thick
+ 1 teaspoon salt
+ 1/2 to 1 teaspoon ground chipotle chile, to taste
+ 2 teaspoons extra-virgin olive oil
+ 1/4 cup fresh lime juice
+ 1/2 cup chopped fresh cilantro or mint
+ 2 avocados, cut in half, pitted, flesh scooped out and mashed with a little lime juice and salt
+ Simply Tomato Salsa (page 50), Green Salsa (page 52), or jarred salsa

The Truth About Tortillas

When the label reads *flour tortillas*, you can bet that that flour is white flour, and often a long list of unpronounceable ingredients and hydrogenated oils follows. Look for the words *no preservatives or additives*, *100 percent whole-wheat flour* (if it's not 100 percent whole wheat it will often contain white flour as well), or *100 percent corn flour*, and a short ingredient list. Refrigerated or frozen tortillas tend to have more wholesome ingredients than those found on the shelf. And your fast-food tortillas are most likely filled with those unpronounceable ingredients and unhealthy oils, so steer clear of those if you can!

Wrapper options

+ 8 corn or other whole-grain tortillas, warmed
+ 8 tender cabbage leaves
+ 8 very thin peeled turnip slices

1. In a large bowl, combine the fish, salt, and chile powder and toss to coat well, taking care not to crumble the fish.

2. Heat the oil in a large nonstick skillet over medium-high heat. Add the fish and sauté until just cooked through, 3 to 4 minutes, stirring often. Remove from the heat and stir in the lime juice. Transfer the fish to a serving bowl and stir in the cilantro.

3. To serve, lay out your wrappers, top with some fish (scoop it out with a slotted spoon to avoid getting your wrappers soggy with the juices), and finish with avocado and a spoonful of salsa.

Shrimp in Carrot Sauce

SERVES 4

Simple dining at its finest, and easiest! White tablecloth optional.

- 1 pound large shrimp, peeled and deveined
- 1 lemon, quartered
- 2 cups carrot juice
- 1/2 teaspoon salt, or to taste
- 1/8 teaspoon ground cinnamon
- 1/8 teaspoon ground nutmeg
- Pinch of ground cloves
- Pinch of ground cayenne
- 2 tablespoons unsalted butter
- 2 bunches baby bok choy, thinly sliced
- 1 tablespoon fresh lemon juice

1. Fill a large saucepan with water and add the lemon quarters. Bring to a boil and add the shrimp. Cook until just cooked through and opaque throughout, 1 to 2 minutes. Drain and run cold water over the shrimp to stop the cooking.

2. Meanwhile, in a medium saucepan, combine the carrot juice, salt, cinnamon, nutmeg, cloves, and cayenne. Place over medium-high heat and bring to a simmer; simmer until reduced to about 1/2 cup, about 20 minutes. Stir in the butter until melted. Add the shrimp and bok choy, cover, and cook for 1 to 2 minutes, lifting the lid once or twice to stir, until the shrimp is warmed through and the bok choy is wilted. Add the lemon juice. Taste and season with more lemon juice, salt, and/or pepper if needed.

Shrimp Fra Diavolo

SERVES 4

Here I've greened up this classic Italian entrée by boosting it with a generous amount of Swiss chard. If Swiss chard isn't available, try using spinach or another tender leafy green. Note that shrimp fra diavolo is heavy on the garlic and red pepper; milder tastes can reduce the amount of either or both. Don't skimp on the Parmesan, though, as it really ties the flavors together.

+ 2½ tablespoons extra-virgin olive oil
+ 1 pound medium to large shrimp, peeled and deveined
+ 1 to 1½ teaspoons red pepper flakes
+ 1 teaspoon salt, or to taste
+ 8 garlic cloves, minced
+ 1/2 teaspoon onion powder
+ 1/2 cup dry white wine or low-sodium vegetable or chicken stock (see the recipe on page 154 or use store-bought)
+ 1 (28-ounce) can no-salt-added diced tomatoes, including juices
+ 2 teaspoons apple cider vinegar, or to taste
+ 1 teaspoon honey
+ 1 bunch Swiss chard, stems removed, leaves torn into pieces
+ 1/4 cup finely chopped fresh parsley
+ 1 pound whole-grain linguine or spaghetti
+ Grated Parmesan cheese for serving

1. Bring a large pot of water to a boil.

2. Meanwhile, in a large bowl, combine the shrimp with 1 tablespoon of the oil, 1/2 teaspoon of the red pepper flakes, and 1/2 teaspoon salt.

3. Heat a large skillet over medium-high heat. Add the shrimp to the skillet in a single layer and cook without moving them, until the bottoms start to color, about 30 seconds. Quickly remove from the heat, turn the shrimp using tongs, and cook for another 30 seconds or so. Remove the shrimp from the pan to a bowl.

4. Add the remaining 1½ tablespoons oil, the garlic, and onion powder to the pan and sauté, stirring, until the garlic is lightly colored, about 2 minutes, adding a tiny bit of water if the garlic starts to stick to the pan. Add the remaining 1/2 teaspoon red pepper flakes and the wine and stir until the wine is mostly evaporated, about 5 minutes. Add the tomatoes, vinegar, honey, and the remaining 1/2 teaspoon salt, bring to a simmer, then reduce the heat to low and cook for about 20 minutes, until the sauce thickens slightly.

5. While the sauce simmers, add the linguine to the pot and cook according to the package directions for al dente. Drain.

6. Add the chard leaves to the sauce by the handful and stir each handful until it is wilted. Add the shrimp and heat until cooked through, 1 to 2 minutes. Stir in the parsley.

7. Divide the linguine among bowls and serve, topped with the shrimp, chard, and sauce. Don't forget the Parmesan!

Seared Scallops Perfected

SERVES 4

Many of us think of scallops as a special-occasion restaurant dish, but guess what—it's simple to sear them to perfection at home, making them an option for any day of the week, pan to plate in under five minutes.

It's easy to overcook scallops; a few seconds too long takes them from tender to rubbery, but not if you follow three rules—1) cook them in a super-hot pan, 2) take them out of the pan just when they turn translucent, and 3) serve them the instant they come out of the pan.

+ 12 large scallops, cleaned
+ Sea salt and freshly ground black pepper
+ 1 to 2 tablespoons extra-virgin olive oil
+ Squeeze of fresh lemon or lime juice

1. Place the scallops on a paper towel–lined plate, pat the tops dry with a paper towel, and season them with salt and pepper to taste on the top side.

2. Heat the oil in a large skillet over high heat until super-hot. Quickly add the scallops to the pan seasoned side down, season the tops with salt and pepper to taste, and cook for 1 to 2 minutes, until well browned around the edges and on the bottom, then flip them in the order that you placed them in the pan (to

Step It Up!
Immediately after plating the scallops, add a splash of white wine and a pat of butter to the pan. Swirl the pan to melt the butter and drizzle over the scallops.

ensure even cooking—this is important) and cook on the second side for about 1 minute, until just cooked through (just going from translucent to opaque inside). Squeeze a little lemon juice on the scallops just as they are finishing cooking.

3. Quickly remove from the pan to a new paper towel–lined plate to absorb excess oil, then transfer to serving plates and serve immediately, with your choice of accompaniments.

Serving Companions
Corn and Red Onion Salsa (page 54)
Anytime Vegetables (page 101)
Puttanesca Salsa (page 53)
Everyday Green Salad All Dressed Up (page 78)
Summer Squash Ribbon Salad (page 91)
Brussels Sprouts Confetti (page 105)
Garlicky Butternut Squash Mash (page 106)
Green Beans with Toasted Coconut (page 104)
Drizzled with pesto (page 48)
Whole grain of your choice (pages 111 to 122)

Fish Fillets
Three Simple Ways

SERVES 4

As people transition to a healthy diet, they tend to favor chicken but miss out on a couldn't-be-simpler any-day dinner option: fish.

Use any type of fish, from bass to yellowtail, and be aware that fish doesn't have to break your budget—amid your many choices you'll likely find one that's on sale, often half the price of other options. Going for frozen is another excellent strategy (fish that's been frozen works best for steaming or roasting rather than searing because it tends to retain water). When using frozen fish, rinse the fillets briefly under very cold water until the surface glaze is melted, then pat dry with paper towels before cooking.

- 4 (6-ounce) fish fillets, any remaining bones removed
- Salt and freshly ground black pepper
- Extra-virgin olive oil cooking spray if searing or roasting
- Lettuce or Napa cabbage leaves if steaming
- Lemon wedges for serving

To sear the fish:

Heat a large sauté pan over medium-high heat until very hot. Season the fish with salt and pepper. Spray the pan with cooking spray and add the fish fillets to the pan skin side down, pressing a few times on the fillets with a spatula for the first 30 seconds to prevent the fish from curling. Cook until almost all the way cooked through (you'll see a white line rise up the fillets as they cook; you want that white line to almost reach the top of the fish), 3 to 5 minutes. Flip the fish and cook for about 20 seconds, until the fish is just cooked through.

To steam the fish:

Fill a large saucepan with about 1 inch of water and bring to a simmer over medium heat. Line a steamer insert or colander with wide lettuce or Napa cabbage leaves. Place the steamer insert into the pan (make sure water doesn't touch the bottom) and lay the fillets onto the vegetables. Cover and steam for about 3 minutes for fresh fish, 5 to 7 minutes for frozen fish, until the fish is just cooked through. Season with salt and pepper to taste.

To roast the fish:

Preheat the oven to 450°F and spray a baking dish with cooking spray. Place the fillets on the dish and spray the tops of the fish with cooking spray. Place in the oven and roast for 5 minutes, then open the oven door and season with salt and pepper. Continue to roast for about 10 minutes, until the fish is just cooked through.

Serve your fish with lemon wedges and your choice of accompaniments.

Grilled Fish Packets

Back when I was a struggling and starved-for-time but hungry-for-brain-food medical school student, this is how I'd make my fish:

1. Defrost fish fillets as above.
2. Spray the dull side of a large square of aluminum foil with extra-virgin olive oil cooking spray.
3. Place a fish fillet in the center, skin side down (one square for each fillet).
4. Drizzle the top of the fish with olive oil, season with spices, salt, and pepper, and load the packet with veggies—any type you like that cooks quickly such as mushrooms and peppers.
5. Seal and throw on the grill for about 10 minutes, remove, unfold (be mindful of the hot steam!), and serve—an impressive presentation with very little effort!

Serving Companions

Corn and Red Onion Salsa (page 54)

Anytime Vegetables (page 101)

Puttanesca Salsa (page 53)

Everyday Green Salad All Dressed Up (page 78)

Summer Squash Ribbon Salad (page 91)

Brussels Sprouts Confetti (page 105)

Garlicky Butternut Squash Mash (page 106)

Green Beans with Toasted Coconut (page 104)

Drizzled with pesto (page 48)

Wrapped in a whole-grain tortilla

Whole grain of your choice (pages 111 to 122)

Poached Salmon Perfected Ⓢ

SERVES 2

If you're intimidated by fish, here's a great recipe for beginners. This method avoids the oil of traditional pan cooking, just the thing for days when you're keeping closer track of your calories. How you serve the fish is entirely up to you; I've included ample choices below. Make sure to purchase BPA-free bags to poach your fish in (learn more about why to avoid BPA on page 43).

+ 2 (4-ounce) salmon fillets, any remaining bones removed
+ Salt and freshly ground black pepper
+ Extra-virgin olive oil
+ Lemon wedges

1. Season the salmon with salt and pepper to taste and place each fillet in a small heavy-duty zip-top bag. Roll the bag around the fish, pressing to remove all the air, then seal the bag.

2. Fill a large, deep skillet with water and bring to a bare simmer. Using tongs, lower the salmon bags into the water with the seal of the bag facing down and cook until just firm, 4 to 5 minutes for medium-rare, a minute or so longer for medium. Cut open the bags and roll the fillets with their juices out onto serving plates.

3. Serve with a drizzle of oil and the lemon wedges alongside, along with your choice of accompaniments.

Spinach Curry with Chickpeas

SERVES 2 TO 3 AS A MAIN OR 4 TO 6 AS A SIDE

This super-quick curry is a fresher, lighter take on the popular saag paneer (spinach and cheese in cream sauce) dishes you'll find on most Indian menus, with chickpeas taking the place of the cheese and a little Greek yogurt added at the end for creaminess. Serve over your whole grain of choice or solo if you're closely watching your carbs today.

- 2 teaspoons extra-virgin olive oil
- 1 medium red onion, chopped
- 2 garlic cloves, minced
- 2 teaspoons minced peeled fresh ginger
- 3/4 teaspoon ground cumin
- 3/4 teaspoon ground coriander
- 1/4 teaspoon ground turmeric
- 1/4 teaspoon ground cayenne, or to taste
- 1 (14-ounce) can no-salt-added diced tomatoes
- 1 (15-ounce) can no-salt-added chickpeas, drained and rinsed, or 1½ cups cooked dried chickpeas
- 1 teaspoon salt, or to taste
- 8 ounces baby spinach leaves
- 1/3 cup plain Greek yogurt

 Time-saver: Used jarred minced garlic and ginger, or if you find your way into an Indian grocery, pick up a jar of ginger-garlic paste. This will save you the trouble of chopping the ginger and garlic in one shot.

1. Heat the oil in a large sauté pan over medium-high heat. Add the onion and cook, stirring often, until softened and starting to brown, about 5 minutes. Add the garlic and ginger and cook for 2 minutes; add a tiny bit of water to the pan if the mixture starts to stick. Add the cumin, coriander, turmeric, and cayenne and cook, stirring, until aromatic, about 1 minute, again adding a tiny bit of water to the pan if the mixture starts to stick.

2. Add the tomatoes and stir to release any browned bits from the bottom of the pan. Add the chickpeas and salt and bring to a simmer. Cover, reduce the heat, and simmer for 15 minutes. Uncover the pan, increase the heat to medium-high, and add the spinach by the handful, stirring to wilt each addition. When all the spinach is added and wilted, stir in the yogurt just until heated through (don't cook it for too long or it can start to separate) and serve.

Chicken Curry

SERVES 6

This satisfying everyday curry is a great entry into Indian cooking and something you'll likely want to put into your dinner rotation. I call for dark meat because it's deliciously satisfying and allows you to spend more time cooking the spices into the meat without fear of it drying out. To trim calories, you could substitute chicken breast and reduce the cooking time to 10 minutes, or you could simply serve the dark meat curry in smaller portions, reduce the amount of rice you serve it with, or skip the rice entirely. Just know that you have options!

See page 147 to educate yourself about the Indian pantry and page 146 for a time-saver tip for making your curry.

+ 1 tablespoon extra-virgin olive oil
+ 1 large red onion, chopped
+ 1 tablespoon minced fresh ginger
+ 3 garlic cloves, minced
+ 1½ teaspoons ground coriander
+ 1½ teaspoons ground cumin
+ 1/4 teaspoon ground cayenne, or to taste
+ 1/4 teaspoon ground turmeric
+ 2 pounds dark meat chicken, trimmed of fat and cut into 1-inch pieces
+ 3/4 cup canned no-salt-added or fresh diced tomatoes
+ 1½ teaspoons salt, or to taste
+ 1/4 cup plain Greek yogurt (optional)
+ 1 cup chopped fresh cilantro
+ Brown rice for serving (optional)

1. Heat the oil in a large sauté pan over medium-high heat. Add the onion and cook, stirring often, until well browned (really brown it, more than you might think—this makes a big difference in flavor), about 7 minutes. Add the ginger and garlic and cook, stirring, for 2 minutes; add a tiny bit of water if the mixture starts to stick to the bottom of the pan. Add the coriander, cumin, cayenne, and turmeric and cook, stirring, for about 1 minute, until aromatic, again adding a tiny bit of water if the mixture starts to stick.

2. Add the chicken, stir well to coat the meat with the spices, and cook for 5 minutes, adding a little water once again if the mixture starts to stick. Add 2 tablespoons water and stir to release any browned bits from the bottom of the pan, then add the tomatoes and salt. Bring to a simmer, then reduce the heat to low, cover, and simmer for about 20 minutes, until the chicken is cooked through and coated with the sauce. Turn off the heat and stir in the yogurt, if using, to heat it through.

3. Stir in the cilantro and serve over brown rice if you like.

Add Veggies!
When the curry is close to completed, add a handful of tender leafy greens such as spinach or Swiss chard and stir until wilted, or add green beans cut into 1-inch pieces 5 to 10 minutes before your curry is done.

Spicy Chicken Stew

SERVES 8

Quite simply, this is spicy food at its best. As a bonus, the thermogenic effects of the chiles will help you burn some calories as you chew!

+ 2 teaspoons extra-virgin olive oil
+ 2 pounds boneless chicken thighs, trimmed of excess fat and cut into 1-inch pieces
+ 1 medium onion, chopped
+ 3 medium bell peppers (a mix of colors), cored, seeded, and chopped
+ 2 or 3 jalapeño chiles, seeded and chopped
+ 2 teaspoons minced fresh ginger
+ 2 garlic cloves, minced
+ 1 large tomato, chopped
+ 1 teaspoon salt, or to taste
+ Brown rice or other whole grain, for serving (optional)

Make Ahead: The dish keeps well—for up to 4 days—and since it's so easy to make, I've bumped the servings up to 8, enough for dinner plus lunches to bring to work.

Chiles, a staple in cuisines throughout the world, have been honored for their medicinal value for well over 2,000 years. Chiles offer various nutrients, particularly vitamin C (one green chile provides more than 100 milligrams, more than the daily requirement), but chiles are particularly lauded for their spicy compounds, most notably capsaicin. Capsaicin is an anti-inflammatory and has been used in treating pain and neuropathy, both topically and internally; it also aids in the metabolism of fats, helps to balance blood sugar, and increases blood circulation, making chiles an excellent ally in cardiovascular health.

1. Heat the oil in a large sauté pan over medium-high heat. Add the chicken and leave for about 3 minutes without stirring (so the fat releases from the chicken and the meat doesn't stick to the pan), then stir and cook, stirring often, until the chicken is no longer pink, about 10 minutes.

2. Add the onion, bell peppers, jalapeño, ginger, and garlic and cook, stirring often, for about 10 minutes, until the vegetables are softened. Add the tomato and salt, then reduce the heat to medium and cook for about 10 more minutes, until the chicken and vegetables are very tender and the flavors have melded.

3. Serve immediately, over brown rice or another grain of choice if you like.

Add Veggies!
Stir in a handful of frozen peas or carrots during the last 5 minutes of cooking.

Crispy Roasted Chicken

SERVES 4

The crispiest and most tender chicken is one that's quick roasted at a high temperature. See the following recipes to make the most of your roast.

+ 1 (3-pound) whole chicken, trimmed of excess fat
+ 1 to 2 tablespoons extra-virgin olive oil
+ 1 teaspoon dried herbs such as rosemary, thyme, sage, or oregano, or a combination
+ Salt and freshly ground black pepper

1. Preheat the oven to 500°F. Line a roasting pan with aluminum foil and set a wire rack into the pan.

2. In a small bowl, combine the oil, herbs, and salt and pepper to taste and set aside.

3. Rinse the chicken and pat thoroughly dry with paper towels. Place the chicken breast side down on the rack, place in the oven, and roast for about 20 minutes. Baste with some of the seasoned olive oil, then turn the bird breast side up, baste with more oil, and return to the oven for 5 to 7 minutes, until lightly browned.

4. Reduce the oven temperature to 325°F, baste again, and roast until an instant-read thermometer inserted into the thickest part of the thigh registers 165°F, about 30 minutes more.

5 Remove from the oven and tilt the chicken so the juices from the cavity drip into the pan. Remove from the pan, place on a platter or carving board, and let rest for 5 minutes before carving and serving. Serve with or without the pan juices.

Now What? Make Chicken Stock!

Dinner's done and you've shredded what's left of the chicken for tomorrow's chicken salad (see pages 156 to 158), making double duty of your roast. Don't stop there! With a tiny bit more effort—no more than tossing the bones into a pot, adding water, and watching the pot every now and then—you've got homemade chicken stock (see pages 154 to 155). And if you have a slow cooker, it's even easier. If you don't have the whole 2 to 3 pounds of bones handy, make a half batch, or gather up your bones in the freezer and make stock once you've got enough saved up—don't worry about exact amounts.

Chicken Stock

MAKES ABOUT 3½ QUARTS

Homemade stock contains collagen and gelatin, great for hair, nails, and healthy bones as we grow and as we age, and it's loaded with highly absorbable minerals, including calcium, magnesium, and phosphorus. Homemade stock will save you money over boxed or canned (it's basically free, as it makes use of bones you would have otherwise tossed), puts you in charge of how much if any salt you add, and it makes any recipe you use it in taste better. Note that the vinegar helps bring out minerals from the bones and into the stock. If boxed or canned stock is more your speed, see page 64 on how to choose a quality brand.

+ 2 to 3 pounds chicken bones
+ 4 quarts cold water
+ Chopped vegetables: a couple carrots, an onion, a couple celery stalks, a couple unpeeled garlic cloves, whatever you have handy (optional)
+ 2 tablespoons vinegar (any type)
+ Salt (optional)

1. Place the bones in a large stockpot. Add the water and bring just to a boil, then boil for 5 minutes, skimming any foam from the top of the pot. Add the vegetables, if using, the vinegar, and salt to taste, if using, cover, reduce the heat to very low, and cook at a bare simmer for 12 hours. Alternatively, combine all the ingredients in a slow cooker, turn it to low, and cook for 12 to 24 hours.

2. Remove the bones with tongs or a slotted spoon, then strain the stock through a fine-mesh strainer lined with cheesecloth into a heatproof bowl. Use immediately, or cool, pour into containers, and store in the refrigerator for up to 1 week or in the freezer for up to 3 months. If you like, you can reuse the bones two or three times more to make multiple batches of stock.

Getting Creative with Chicken Salad

Here are three flavor-packed ways to turn last night's roast (page 152) or leftover poached chicken (page 75) into chicken salad for lunch.

Orange, Fennel, and Rosemary Chicken Salad

MAKES ABOUT 4 CUPS

+ 4 cups shredded cooked chicken (page 75 or 152)
+ 1/2 cup thinly sliced fennel
+ 1/4 cup chopped fennel fronds
+ 1 to 2 tablespoons extra-virgin olive oil
+ 1/4 cup freshly squeezed orange juice
+ 1½ teaspoons grated orange zest
+ 2 teaspoons minced fresh rosemary
+ 1/4 to 1/2 teaspoon salt, to taste
+ 1/4 teaspoon freshly ground black pepper

In a large bowl, combine all the ingredients and stir well to fully incorporate. Serve as a salad atop a bed of lettuce or in the sandwich wrapper of your choice.

Deconstructed Pesto Chicken Salad

+ 4 cups shredded cooked chicken (page 75 or 152)
+ 2 to 3 tablespoons extra-virgin olive oil
+ 1 cup packed fresh basil
+ 1/4 cup toasted pine nuts
+ 2 to 3 tablespoons grated Parmesan cheese
+ 1 tablespoon grated lemon zest
+ 3 tablespoons fresh lemon juice, or to taste
+ 1/4 to 1/2 teaspoon salt, to taste
+ 1/4 teaspoon cracked black pepper

In a large bowl, combine all the ingredients and stir well to fully incorporate. Serve as a salad atop a bed of lettuce or in the sandwich wrapper of your choice.

Broccoli Chicken Salad

MAKES ABOUT 4 CUPS

+ 3 cups shredded cooked chicken (page 75 or 152)
+ 1½ cups cooked or raw broccoli florets
+ 1/4 to 1/3 cup olive oil mayonnaise
+ 3 tablespoons finely chopped shallot or red onion
+ 1 teaspoon Dijon-style mustard
+ 2 tablespoons fresh herbs, such as dill, cilantro, mint, parsley, or a combination
+ 1 tablespoon fresh lemon juice, or to taste

In a large bowl, combine all the ingredients and stir well to fully incorporate. Serve as a salad atop a bed of lettuce or in the sandwich wrapper of your choice.

Super-Quick Tuna Melt

SERVES 1

Perfect for times when it seems there's no time at all for dinner. If you have two minutes, you have a tasty meal! You might try substituting canned salmon for the tuna to change things up; vegetarians can swap canned beans (heat them in the microwave with the cheese), Southwestern-Style Black Bean Dip (page 42), Zucchini Hummus (page 44), or Pumpkin Seed Salsa (page 45) for the tuna. Another option: mix hummus and olive oil in with the tuna and place it over whole-grain toast for an open-faced tuna sandwich.

+ 1 whole-grain tortilla (see page 135 on choosing)
+ 2 to 4 tablespoons shredded Jack or other cheese
+ 1 (3- to 5-ounce) can tuna packed in water, drained, or predrained packet
+ Handful of spinach or lettuce
+ Drizzle of extra-virgin olive oil
+ Salt and freshly ground black pepper

Place the tortilla on a microwave-safe plate. Sprinkle with the cheese and microwave on high for 20 seconds, or until the cheese melts. Top with the tuna, followed by the spinach. Drizzle with a little olive oil, season with salt and pepper to taste, and serve.

Quicksadillas

MAKES 6 QUESADILLAS

Thus named because you've already got the chicken from leftovers and the zucchini cooks right into the tortillas, making quick work of dinner. To keep your batches warm while the remaining cook, place quicksadillas on a baking sheet in a preheated 200°F oven as they come off the pan.

To turn your quicksadillas vegetarian, substitute black beans for the chicken. See page 135 on choosing the most health-supportive tortillas.

+ 2 small zucchinis (about 8 ounces)
+ 1/4 teaspoon salt
+ 1 cup shredded leftover chicken
+ 1/2 cup (2 ounces) grated Jack cheese
+ 2 scallions, chopped
+ 1/4 red bell pepper, cored, seeded, and finely chopped (optional)
+ Couple dashes of hot sauce, or to taste
+ 6 (6-inch) 100 percent corn or other whole-grain tortillas (see page 135 on how to choose)
+ Guacamole (page 59) and/or salsa (page 50 to 54), for serving

> ### One-Minute Quicksadillas
>
> If you're truly time crunched, it's OK to keep it really simple. Lay a whole-grain tortilla flat on a microwave-safe plate and top with a few spoonfuls of precooked black beans (and/or leftover chicken) and sprinkle some grated cheese on top if you like. Microwave on high for about 1 minute, until the cheese is melted. Add guacamole, salsa, a few dashes of hot sauce, and spinach for a little health boost. Fold in half. Voila. Who said a quickie couldn't be great?!

1. Cut the stem ends from the zucchini and grate the zucchini on the large holes of a box grater. In a colander, toss the grated zucchini with the salt using your hands and squeeze the zucchini to remove most of its liquid. Remove more liquid by patting it with a paper towel.

2. In a large bowl, combine the zucchini, chicken, cheese, scallions, red pepper, if using, and hot sauce. Taste the mixture and add more salt and/or hot sauce to taste if needed.

3. Heat a large cast-iron or nonstick skillet over medium heat. Working one at a time, warm the tortillas in the skillet until pliable, about 10 seconds per side, then transfer to a work surface. Scoop one-sixth (about 1/4 cup) of the chicken on top of each tortilla and fold in half over the filling.

4. Spray the skillet with cooking spray. Add 3 of the quicksadillas and spray the tops with cooking spray. Cook until lightly browned on the bottom and the cheese is melted, about 2 minutes. Flip and brown the other side, about 2 minutes longer. Repeat with the remaining quicksadillas, adding more cooking spray to the pan as you go. Serve with a generous dollop of guacamole and/or salsa on the side.

Mexi Chicken Bowl

SERVES 1

On the busiest of days, the microwave can make the difference between a healthy at-home meal and a trip through the drive-thru. This bowl is quicker than the latter and a wholesome upgrade to typical Mexican fare. Vegetarians can substitute cubed firm tofu for the chicken or skip it altogether. If there's any guacamole in the fridge, a little bit of that can go on top as well or can be added in place of the cheese.

+ 1/4 cup cooked brown rice (page 112) or quinoa (page 118) (optional)
+ 1/2 cup shredded cooked chicken (page 75 or 152)
+ 1/2 cup no-salt-added canned black beans, drained and rinsed
+ 1/4 cup Simply Tomato Salsa (page 50) or jarred salsa
+ 2 to 4 tablespoons shredded cheddar or pepper Jack cheese
+ Handful of spinach or lettuce
+ Dollop of plain Greek yogurt

Layer the brown rice, if using, chicken, beans, salsa, and cheese in a microwave-safe bowl. Cover and microwave on high for about 1 minute, until heated through and the cheese is melted. Top with the lettuce and yogurt and serve.

Chunky Chili

SERVES 8

While the ingredients list may seem long, the method is easy, no more than chopping, sautéing, and cooking everything together to meld into this satisfying stew. If you're closely watching your carbs, try wrapping your chili in steamed kale leaves. If you're not up for peeling and cutting up a squash (not always an easy task), feel free to use pre-cubed squash, which you'll find in the produce aisle.

- 1 tablespoon extra-virgin olive oil
- 1 small butternut squash (about 2 pounds), peeled, cut in half, seeds scooped out, cut into 1/2-inch cubes
- 1 yellow onion, chopped
- 1 green bell pepper, cored, seeded, and chopped
- 1 red bell pepper, cored, seeded, and chopped
- 1 jalapeño chile, seeded and minced
- 2 garlic cloves, minced
- 1 tablespoon ground cumin
- 1 teaspoon dried oregano
- 1/2 teaspoon ground cinnamon
- 1 (15-ounce) can no-salt-added diced tomatoes with juices
- 1 cup low-sodium vegetable or chicken stock (see the recipe on page 154 or use store-bought) or water
- 2 (15-ounce) cans no-salt-added black beans, drained and rinsed
- 1 tablespoon apple cider vinegar

Continues ▶

- ✚ 1 to 2 teaspoons salt, to taste
- ✚ Brown rice or another grain (pages 111 to 122), whole-grain tortillas, or steamed kale leaves for serving
- ✚ Topping options: shredded Jack cheese, sliced avocado, sliced scallions, chopped cilantro leaves, plain Greek yogurt

1. Heat the oil in a large saucepan over medium-high heat. Add the squash and cook, stirring occasionally, until lightly browned, 5 to 7 minutes. Add the onion, peppers, and jalapeño and cook until softened, about 10 minutes. Add the garlic and cook for 2 minutes. Add the cumin, oregano, and cinnamon and cook until aromatic, about 1 minute.

2. Add the tomatoes, stock, beans, vinegar, and salt and cook, stirring occasionally, until the squash is softened, about 15 minutes. Mash the beans and squash with a potato masher or wooden spoon to your desired chunkiness. Spoon into bowls and serve over brown rice or another grain, tortillas, or steamed kale leaves, with your choice of toppings.

Variation:

Chipotle Black Bean and Butternut Squash Chili: Omit the jalapeño and add 3 chopped canned chipotle chiles in adobo sauce when you add the stock.

 Make Ahead: Chili freezes well. Store it in freezer containers; transfer a container to the refrigerator the night before or in the morning and it will be thawed and ready to heat by dinnertime.

Instant Meatballs with Yogurt Sauce

SERVES 4

Studies have shown that people who eat yogurt are closer to their ideal weight than those who don't, so if you haven't had a bowlful for breakfast, why not try it as a savory sauce for dinner? Vary the type of sausage you use—from spicy Italian to apple to chorizo—to change up the dish.

Sausage

+ 1 pound loose sausage or sausage links, meat removed from casing
+ Extra-virgin olive oil cooking spray

Cucumber-Tomato Yogurt Sauce

+ 1 cup plain yogurt
+ 1/2 small cucumber, peeled, seeded, and minced (about 1/3 cup)
+ 1 small tomato, cored, seeded, and chopped
+ 2 teaspoons fresh lemon juice, or to taste
+ 1/4 cup chopped fresh parsley
+ 1/4 teaspoon salt, or to taste
+ 1/4 teaspoon freshly ground black pepper, or to taste
+ Brown rice or another whole grain (pages 111 to 122), or lettuce or Napa cabbage leaves for serving

Continues ▶

1. Make the meatballs: Preheat the oven to 400°F. Line a baking sheet with parchment paper or aluminum foil and spray with cooking spray.

2. Place the sausage in a large bowl. Form the mixture into about 12 equal-size balls measuring about 1½ inches each. Place the meatballs on the prepared baking sheet and spray with a little more cooking spray. Bake for about 25 minutes, turning once about halfway through cooking, until the meatballs are browned and when you cut into one, you see that the meat inside is no longer pink.

3. Make the sauce: Put the yogurt in a large serving bowl and whisk it to give it a smooth consistency. Stir in the remaining ingredients; taste and adjust the seasonings with more lemon juice and/or salt and pepper if needed.

4. As soon as the meatballs come out of the oven, stir them into the yogurt sauce. Taste and adjust the seasonings with salt and lemon juice if needed and serve.

Variation:

Tomato Yogurt Sauce: Omit the cucumber and double up on the tomato.

 Make Ahead: Roll up a mess of meatballs and freeze them before baking; thaw and bake when you're looking for a quick meal.

Beef and Broccoli Stir-Fry

SERVES 4

Homemade stir-fries are about a million times more healthful than those you'll get from your corner Chinese takeout. Less oil, salt, and sugar—and since you're in charge, you get to load up on the vegetables, turning this former junk food into a good-for-you food. Tip: Don't forget to use the leaves from the broccoli—they are just as nutritious and tasty as the florets.

- 2 tablespoons fresh lime juice
- 1 tablespoon low-sodium soy sauce
- 2 teaspoons rice vinegar
- 2 teaspoons honey or maple syrup
- 2 garlic cloves, pressed through a garlic press
- 1/4 to 1/2 teaspoon red pepper flakes, to taste
- 1 tablespoon unrefined sesame oil or extra-virgin olive oil
- 1 pound sirloin steak, trimmed of excess fat and cut diagonally across the grain into 1/4-inch strips
- 1 large bunch broccoli, cut into small florets, including leaves
- 2 teaspoons cornstarch whisked into 2 tablespoons water to dissolve it
- Brown rice or lettuce or Napa cabbage leaves for serving
- 2 tablespoons toasted sesame seeds or chopped roasted peanuts

1. In a small bowl, whisk together the lime juice, soy sauce, vinegar, honey, garlic, and red pepper flakes. Set aside.

Continues ▶

What's Your Beef? Grass Fed Is Best

In an ideal world, look for grass-fed or pasture-raised meats and meats free of hormones and antibiotics. In *The Doctor's Diet* I mentioned a 2011 study published in the *British Journal of Nutrition* that bears repeating: this study found that subjects who ate grass-fed meat for just four weeks increased their levels of omega-3 fatty acids while decreasing their levels of pro-inflammatory fatty acids. When animals eat grass, they get more omega-3s in their diet—just as we do when we eat our greens—so it intuitively makes sense. Grass-fed beef has also been found to be lower in total fat and higher in beta-carotene, vitamin E, the B vitamins thiamin and riboflavin, and the minerals calcium, magnesium, and potassium.

Consider buying meat from a local farmer so you know where it's coming from and how it was raised; you might even give wild game a try if it's available. If cost is an issue, consider serving smaller, higher quality portions and supplement with other less pricey protein sources such as beans, whole grains, and nuts.

2. Heat the oil in a large skillet over medium-high heat. Add the beef and stir-fry until almost cooked through, about 2 minutes. Remove the beef to a bowl and set aside. Add the broccoli to the pan along with 1/4 cup water, cover, bring to a simmer, then reduce the heat to medium and cook until just barely tender, 2 to 3 minutes.

3. Return the beef to the pan, add the marinade, and cook for 1 minute, then add the cornstarch mixture and cook for another minute or so, stirring constantly, until the sauce thickens and coats the beef and broccoli. Serve over brown rice or in lettuce leaf cups, topped with the sesame seeds.

Very Veggie Burgers

MAKES 6 BURGERS

I grew up in the Midwest, where the term veggie burger *was considered an oxymoron, but this recipe changed my attitude on the concept of what a burger can be. For all you carnivores out there—I encourage you to give it a try! Making it is a little more involved than putting together a typical beef burger, but I think you'll find it worth the added bit of effort.*

+ 1 recipe cooked quinoa (page 118)
+ 1½ cups finely chopped kale leaves
+ 1 (15-ounce) can no-salt-added cannellini beans, drained and rinsed
+ 1/2 cup grated Parmesan cheese
+ 2 teaspoons low-sodium soy sauce, or to taste
+ 1 teaspoon garlic powder
+ 1 teaspoon onion powder
+ 1/4 teaspoon freshly ground black pepper
+ Salt if needed
+ 1 large egg, beaten
+ Extra-virgin olive oil cooking spray
+ Whole-wheat bun halves or a bed of greens
+ Mustard, ketchup, salsa (pages 50 to 54), pesto (page 48), tahini sauce (page 126), or another condiment

Continues ▶

1. Preheat the oven to 400°F and line a baking sheet with parchment or waxed paper.

2. Cook the quinoa as directed on page 118. Just after you turn off the heat, add the kale (don't stir it in), return the cover, and let steam for 10 minutes. Stir the kale into the quinoa, then add the beans and mash them in using a potato masher until mostly mashed with some chunks remaining. Add the cheese, soy sauce, garlic powder, onion powder, and pepper. Taste and adjust the seasonings, adding salt to taste if needed. Cool to room temperature, then stir in the egg to fully incorporate it.

3. Tightly pack the quinoa mixture into heaping 1/2-cup portions (use a measuring cup), then firmly shape the mixture into burger shapes. Place on the prepared baking sheet and spray with cooking spray.

4. Place in the oven and bake for about 30 minutes, flipping them and spraying the second side with cooking spray halfway through baking, until browned and crisp on top.

5. Serve immediately, in buns or over greens if you like, garnished with your choice of toppings.

 Make Ahead: Form the burgers a day ahead and bake when you're ready for dinner, or freeze them and defrost when burgers are on the menu tonight.

LABEL 411

Veggie Burger Busts

Skipping the meat doesn't automatically mean the food you're eating is a health food. Many veggie burger brands contain soy in highly processed form—textured soy protein, soy isolate, or textured vegetable protein—which can be hard on the digestive system. Many contain unhealthy oils too. Read the ingredients list and favor veggie burgers that are based on veggies! (Note: All of the above goes for faux bacon and sausage as well.)

Quinoa: An Ancient Supergrain for Modern Times

Quinoa (pronounced *keen-wah*) has been a staple in the Andean region of South America for thousands of years. It is often referred to as a pseudo-cereal, as it is not technically a grain but is instead a seed from the same vegetable family that includes spinach, chard, and beets. It is unique as a grain in that it proffers all eight essential amino acids, making it a complete protein; it also has a high monounsaturated (good) fat-to-carb ratio. Quinoa is an excellent source of minerals as well as vitamin E and several B vitamins, particularly folate. It's also pretty darn tasty, as its recent rise in popularity can attest to.

Veggie Burger on the Go

SERVES 1

I love making Very Veggie Burgers (page 169) when I've got the time, but when I don't, I'll happily take this shortcut to a quick open-faced veggie burger. It's all about being creative with healthy add-ons from your fridge that make this such an easy but never boring option. This recipe is a reminder that you've always got healthy eating options no matter how busy your day is, and it certainly beats fast food for lunch.

+ 1 frozen prepared veggie burger (see page 171 on choosing)
+ Mustard, ketchup, salsa (pages 50 to 54), pesto (page 48), tahini sauce (page 126), or another condiment
+ 1 whole-grain slice of bread
+ Hummus (pages 44)
+ 1/2 avocado, sliced, or 1/4 cup guacamole (page 59)

Place the veggie burger on a microwave-safe plate and microwave according to the package directions. Spread some mustard or other condiment over the bread, place the veggie burger on top, and top with hummus and avocado and whatever else you can think of that's healthy and in your fridge, whether it's tomatoes, onions, spinach, or pickles. Have fun, be creative, and let your on-the-go veggie burger be a health boost delivery system!

Perfectly Seared Steak

SERVES 4

The key to a perfect steak is patience—if you resist the urge to touch your steak for a few minutes before flipping it, a crust is created and you'll be rewarded with meat that's nicely browned on the outside and just right on the inside. High-quality beef (see page 168) is worth seeking out, and know that when you choose steak for dinner you'll be treating yourself to one of the most absorbable sources of iron you'll find.

Steak

+ 2 (8-ounce) sirloin steaks (about 1½ inches thick), trimmed of excess fat
+ Salt and freshly ground black pepper
+ Extra-virgin olive oil cooking spray
+ 2 tablespoons balsamic vinegar
+ 1/2 teaspoon pure vanilla extract

For serving

+ Brussels Sprouts Confetti (page 105) or any veggie side (pages 97 to 105) or salad (pages 77 to 94) you like
+ Whole grain of choice (pages 111 to 122; optional)

1. Season the steaks with salt and pepper to taste.
2. Lightly spray a large cast-iron skillet or sauté pan with cooking spray and heat over medium-high heat until very hot. Add the steaks and

Continues ▶

leave them without touching for 4 minutes to create a nice crust, then flip them and cook for 4 minutes for medium-rare, a minute or two longer for medium. Place the steaks on a cutting board and let rest for 5 minutes.

3. While the steaks are resting, turn off the heat and add the vinegar and vanilla and let it sizzle for a few seconds (if you are using a cast-iron pan, it will retain a lot of heat and the vinegar may start to dry out; if so, add a little water). Pour the drizzle into a small bowl.

4. To serve, place a bed of confetti or a side on each plate, then thinly slice the steak and arrange on top of the confetti or alongside the side. Drizzle with the vinegar mixture and serve immediately.

 Time-saver: Skip the vinegar and vanilla, and simply serve the steaks in their pan juices.

The New Comfort Food

Food isn't black and white, and following a healthy diet doesn't have to mean dropping entire food categories. Like classic American comfort food, for example: the new comfort food is good for you! Remember the "food as medicine" mantra? Well, now nachos can be medicine, pizza can be medicine, even a burger and fries can be medicine! You can easily eat an unhealthful version of any of these delicious dishes, but by changing up ingredients and amounts, it's just as easy to stay healthy while leaving the table every bit as satisfied. Let's see how!

Nachos

YIELD VARIES

Who says nachos have to be overflowing with unhealthy, processed cheese? Here we don't bake them, as firing up the oven just takes too long when you're hit with a nacho attack. Resist the urge to indulge in that yellow-cheese-covered glop at the local convenience store and try this new approach to nachos, not a set recipe but more of a guideline for assembly. Make as few or as many as you have eaters and include any of the add-on ingredients you have handy in the fridge.

Base

+ 100 percent corn chips (see Label 411 on the next page)
+ Finely shredded romaine lettuce
+ Smoky Black Bean Dip (page 43)

Add-ons

+ Diced avocado
+ Finely chopped seeded tomatoes or salsa (pages 50 to 54)
+ Plain Greek yogurt in place of sour cream
+ Shredded cheese of your choice (optional)
+ Finely chopped scallions or chives

Arrange corn chips on a serving platter. Add a layer of lettuce and top with a spoonful of black bean dip. Finish with your choice of add-ons and serve.

Chip, Chip, Hooray . . . or Dismay?

Not all chips are junk food. What makes most of them unhealthy is the frying and an absurd amount of added sodium. Skip the white potato chips in favor of sweet potato chips, 100 percent corn chips, or 100 percent whole-grain chips that are low in sodium or unsalted, and with few ingredients. Be wary of flavored chips, as they generally contain long, unsavory ingredients lists.

Variations:

Hummus Nachos: Substitute Zucchini Hummus (page 44) for the bean dip.

Pumpkin Seed Salsa Nachos: Substitute Pumpkin Seed Salsa (page 45) for the bean dip.

Sweet Potato Nachos: Substitute Sweet Potato Chips (page 208) for the corn chips.

Cream of Tomato Soup

SERVES 3 TO 4

There's nothing wrong with a little cream, and just a touch is required to fancy up this satisfying soup. Pot to bowl in under 15 minutes, no blending required.

- 2 teaspoons extra-virgin olive oil
- 2 garlic cloves, pressed through a garlic press
- 2 cups low-sodium vegetable or chicken stock (see the recipe on page 54 or use store-bought)
- 1 (15-ounce) can no-salt-added tomato puree
- 2 tablespoons tomato paste
- 1 teaspoon apple cider vinegar, or to taste
- 1/2 teaspoon salt, or to taste
- 1/4 teaspoon freshly ground black pepper
- 1/4 cup heavy cream
- 1 teaspoon honey if needed
- 2 tablespoons finely chopped fresh basil

Step It Up!
Add more fresh herbs, such as rosemary, mint, or oregano.

1. Heat the oil and garlic in a large saucepan over medium heat until the garlic sizzles and turns light golden, about 2 minutes. Add the stock, tomatoes, tomato paste, vinegar, salt, and pepper, increase the heat to high, and bring to a simmer. Reduce the heat to low, cover, and simmer for 10 minutes.

Tomatoes: A Whole Lot of Lycopene

Generally considered a vegetable, tomatoes are actually a citrus fruit. The tomato was first cultivated by the Aztecs and Incas and later brought to Spain by missionaries and conquistadors.

Tomatoes present an excellent nutrient profile (a great source of vitamins A and C, and even some vitamin E) but have received much attention recently for their phytochemical compounds, principally lycopene. Lycopene has been shown to produce twice as much anti-oxidant activity as beta-carotene and has been noted for preventing heart disease and atherosclerosis and defending against various forms of cancer. Eating vegetables raw or only lightly cooked is often the best way to keep phytonutrients intact and beneficial, but in the case of lycopene, it has been found that cooking tomatoes both concentrates and increases the availability of lycopene.

Note that because of their acidity, tomatoes can break down plastics and even draw impurities like aluminum out of metal, so when buying canned tomatoes it is important to source brands packaged in BPA-free cans (read more about this chemical on page 43).

2. Turn off the heat and stir in the cream until heated through. Taste and adjust the seasonings with more vinegar or the honey if needed. Stir in the basil, spoon into bowls, and serve.

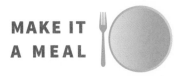

MAKE IT A MEAL Add quinoa or another whole grain, beans, and/or corn, and serve with a hearty salad.

Creamed Spinach

SERVES 4 AS A SIDE

You won't believe how creamy this dairy-free spinach dish is until you try it. Don't be surprised if you find yourself scraping every last bit from the sides of the food processor and scarfing it down as if it were cookie dough instead of spinach! The Step It Up version using baby spinach is even creamier; it's highly recommended if you've got the time.

+ 4 cloves to 1 head garlic, separated into cloves, peeled, and cut in half lengthwise
+ 1/4 cup extra-virgin olive oil
+ 1 (10-ounce) box frozen spinach, thawed
+ 1 tablespoon fresh lemon juice, or to taste
+ 1/4 teaspoon salt, or to taste
+ A few grinds of black pepper

1. In a very small pan (the smaller the better as to fully cover the garlic cloves; a sturdy stainless steel 1-cup measure is a good choice), combine the garlic and oil. Bring to a bare simmer over low heat to poach the garlic for about 10 minutes, until it is soft and lightly golden. If the garlic starts to brown or the oil starts to bubble too fast (this can

Time-saver: Instead of poaching the garlic, pour 2 tablespoons extra-virgin olive oil into a very small saucepan and press 3 garlic cloves through a garlic press into the oil. Heat over low heat until it just comes to a simmer and cook for 30 seconds. Process the garlic oil into the spinach as above.

happen fairly easily), remove the pan from the heat for a few seconds, then return it to the heat.

2. Meanwhile, place the spinach in a strainer and press down on it firmly with your hands to remove as much liquid as possible. (Tip: Use this liquid in place of water in a soup or for grain-making for extra flavor and nutrients.)

3. Place the spinach in a food processor (a mini food processor works especially well for this). Scoop out the garlic from the oil and add the garlic and half of the oil (reserve the remaining garlic-flavored oil to use in your cooking or for another batch of creamed spinach), the lemon juice, salt, and pepper, and puree until creamy, scraping the sides of the machine with a rubber spatula once or twice, as needed, to get at all of it. Taste and adjust the seasonings to your liking. Reheat briefly on the stovetop or in the microwave.

Step It Up!
Instead of frozen spinach, use 1 pound of baby spinach leaves. Place the spinach in a large saucepan, add a couple tablespoons of water, place over medium-high heat, and bring to a boil. Cover and cook, stirring once or twice, for 3 minutes, or until the spinach is completely wilted. (You may need to do this in two batches, depending on the size of your pan.) Drain as you would for the frozen spinach and proceed with the recipe.

Pizza

It's no longer junk food but an irresistible veggie delivery system! When you stick to thin crust pizza, America's favorite comfort food becomes an opportunity to enjoy any number of healthy toppings. Load 'em up!

When shopping for pizza crust, go for whole wheat and the thinnest you can find to keep control of your carbs, and look for a short ingredient list. Many supermarkets also offer frozen whole-grain pizza dough that you thaw, roll out, and bake; these often have more wholesome ingredients. This requires a bit of added effort, but rolling your own is a lot of fun and something the whole family can join in on. A really healthy option is the outrageously addictive Cauliflower Crust pizza—you've got to try it (see recipe on next page). I don't much go for cauliflower on its own, but I love this pizza crust!

+ 1 prepared thin crust whole-wheat pizza shell, rolled-out whole-grain pizza dough, or Cauliflower Crust (page 183)

Topping ideas

+ Broccoli and Mushrooms with Cauliflower Cheese Sauce (recipe follows)
+ Pesto, Roasted Red Peppers, and Cherry Tomatoes (recipe follows)
+ Arugula, Fig, and Goat Cheese (recipe follows)
+ Smoky Black Bean Dip (page 43) topped with chopped tomatoes and sliced green chiles
+ Simply Tomato Sauce (page 56) with shaved zucchini and shaved Parmesan cheese
+ Cucumber Caprese Salad (page 88; add after the pizza is fully baked)

- Chicken Curry (page 148)
- Shredded roasted chicken (page 152) with pesto (page 48) topped with lots of fresh basil
- Creamed Spinach (page 180) topped with tomatoes and grated Parmesan cheese

Bake according to the directions on the package, adding your toppings when indicated, or, if you're making the Cauliflower Crust, following the directions in the sidebar.

Cauliflower Crust

MAKES 1 (9-INCH) CRUST

Cauliflower is the new flour! This crust has made a cauliflower admirer out of me. If you don't tell your guests, I bet they'll never guess what the secret ingredient is.

One crust generally serves two people; since this recipe takes a little extra effort to make, I recommend doubling it to make two crusts, as doing so won't add much extra time.

- 2 (10-ounce) packages frozen cauliflower, thawed (thaw in the refrigerator overnight)

Continues ▶

- 1/4 cup shredded mozzarella cheese
- 1/4 cup shredded Parmesan cheese
- 1 teaspoon garlic powder
- 1/4 teaspoon salt
- 1 large egg

1. Turn a baking sheet upside down, put it in the oven, and preheat the oven to 450°F.

2. Place the cauliflower in a food processor and process to puree it.

3. Wrap the thawed cauliflower in a clean dish towel and wring out as much water as possible (you'll be surprised at how much will come out).

4. Place the cauliflower in a large bowl and add the mozzarella and Parmesan cheeses, the garlic powder, and salt and mix everything together with your hands to combine the ingredients thoroughly. Add the egg and mix it in with your hands.

5. Form the mixture into a round of dough and place it on a sheet of parchment paper. Pat the dough down with your hands to form it into an even 9-inch round crust about 1/4-inch thick with a little indentation around the perimeter to keep the toppings from spilling off the sides.

6. Slide the parchment onto the hot baking sheet and bake for 10 to 12 minutes, until it starts to brown. Remove from the oven. Add your choice of toppings and bake until bubbling, 5 to 7 minutes. Remove from the oven, slice, and serve.

Broccoli and Mushrooms with Cauliflower Cheese Sauce

+ 2 teaspoons extra-virgin olive oil
+ 3 cups sliced mushrooms
+ 1 cup small broccoli florets
+ 1/4 to 1/2 cup cauliflower cheese sauce (page 130)

Heat the oil in a large skillet over medium heat. Add the mushrooms and cook until softened, about 10 minutes. Add the broccoli and cook until crisp-tender, 3 to 5 minutes. Remove from the heat. Spread the sauce over the pizza crust, top with the broccoli and mushrooms, top with a little more sauce if you like, and bake as directed above.

Pesto, Roasted Red Peppers, and Yellow Cherry Tomatoes

+ 2 to 3 tablespoons pesto (page 48)
+ 1/2 cup cherry tomatoes, cut in half
+ 1 roasted red bell pepper, patted dry and cut into strips
+ 1 tablespoon grated cheese of your choice (optional)

Spread the pesto over the crust and arrange the cherry tomatoes and red peppers over the pesto. Top with the cheese, if using, and bake as directed above.

Arugula, Fig, and Goat Cheese Pizza

- 2 dried or fresh figs
- 2 ounces fresh goat cheese, crumbled
- 4 cups (about 2 ounces) arugula leaves
- Extra-virgin olive oil cooking spray
- Balsamic vinegar
- Salt and freshly ground black pepper

If using dried figs, soak them in hot water for 30 minutes to soften, then drain. Arrange the goat cheese and figs over the crust and top with the arugula. Spray with some cooking spray and add a drizzle of vinegar and a sprinkling of salt and pepper. Bake as directed above. If you prefer not to wilt the arugula, toss it with a little oil and vinegar and season with salt and pepper to taste. Bake the pizza crust with the goat cheese and figs, slice it, then add the arugula to individual slices.

Quick Fix
Spinach Lasagna

SERVES 4

This recipe appeared in The Doctor's Diet *(and you might have seen me preparing it on an episode of* The Doctors*), and it became a fast favorite. So many people have told me how it's become a regular in their dinner rotation that I just had to include it again for those of you who might have missed it. Minimal prep, maximum satisfaction, and tasty every time! For those who are gluten-free, substitute brown rice lasagna for the whole wheat.*

+ Extra-virgin olive oil cooking spray
+ 16 ounces cottage cheese
+ 1 (8-ounce bag) fresh spinach
+ 1 large egg
+ 1/4 to 1/2 teaspoon red chile flakes
+ Pinch of salt, or to taste
+ 8 ounces cooked or no-boil whole-wheat lasagna noodles
+ 1 cup Simply Tomato Sauce (page 56) or low-sodium store-bought tomato sauce
+ 1/2 cup shredded mozzarella cheese

1. Preheat the oven to 350°F and spray an 8 by 12–inch baking dish with cooking spray.

2. In a large bowl, combine the cottage cheese, spinach, egg, chile flakes, and salt.

Continues ▶

3. Spread out half of the lasagna noodles on the baking dish. Cover with the cheese-spinach filling and top with the remaining noodles. Pour the sauce over the noodles and sprinkle with the mozzarella cheese.

4. Place in the oven and bake for 45 to 50 minutes, until bubbly and lightly browned on top. Let rest for 5 minutes before slicing and serving.

The New Classic Burger

SERVES 4

The new burger is a healthful burger, with your choice of meat—preferably grass fed (see page 168 to learn more about grass-fed meat)—served open-faced on a whole-grain bun half or on a bed of greens if you're watching your carbs. For a complex-carb companion, serve with Sweet Potato Fries (page 192), or if it's a carb-light night, go for the Zucchini Fries (page 191). Favor ketchup that's free of high-fructose corn syrup.

+ 1 pound lean ground beef, turkey, or buffalo
+ 1/2 teaspoon salt
+ 1/4 teaspoon freshly ground black pepper
+ Whole-grain bun halves or a bed of sautéed kale, spinach, or spring greens
+ Mustard, ketchup, salsa (pages 50 to 54), or your choice of condiments

1. Combine the beef, salt, and pepper in a large bowl and mix gently but thoroughly to combine.

2. Divide the mixture into 4 equal portions and form each into a loose ball. Pat tightly to flatten the meat into a patty about 1/2-inch thick. Press the center of the patties down a little with your fingertips to create an indentation in the center, resulting in edges that are thicker than the center (this keeps your burgers from puffing up as they cook).

3. Heat a large heavy-bottomed skillet, preferably cast-iron, over

Continues ▶

A Buyer's Guide to Ground Meat

On page 168 I talked about the advantages of choosing quality beef; when it comes to ground meat, being choosy is particularly important. Ground meat carries certain risks because rather than being sourced from one animal in one place, it can be an assortment of different grades of meat from random cow parts and even from slaughterhouses thousands of miles apart. About 70 percent of ground beef products contain cheap meat filler. The nutritive value in this type of meat is substantially lower and the risks for *E. coli* contamination are much greater. There is no labeling system in place to indicate the source and processing of ground meat, so the best way to avoid these risks is knowing where your meat comes from—by shopping at a farmers' market, buying your meat from a knowledgeable butcher or direct from the farm, or choosing ground meat labeled "organic." Make it worth the trip for good-quality ground meat by stocking up; it will keep for months in the freezer.

medium-high heat until very hot. Add the patties indentation side up and cook on each side for about 3 minutes for rare, 3½ minutes for medium-rare, 4 minutes for medium, and 5 minutes for well-done. Serve immediately, in buns or over kale if you like, garnished with your choice of toppings.

Zucchini Fries

SERVES 4

Trust me, you won't miss the fried potatoes when you try these. Zucchini bakes till crisp on the outside, tender and juicy on the inside—so satisfying, so easy. If fries are a weakness of yours, you might look into purchasing an air fryer, a countertop machine that "fries" your favorite foods to crispy deliciousness via circulating hot air with minimal or no oil. This recipe easily doubles to fill two baking sheets.

+ Extra-virgin olive oil cooking spray
+ 2 large zucchinis
+ 2 egg whites
+ 1/4 cup whole-wheat breadcrumbs
+ 1/2 teaspoon dried herbs of choice, such as oregano, rosemary, or thyme (optional)
+ Salt and freshly ground black pepper

1. Preheat the oven to 450°F. Spray a baking sheet with cooking spray.
2. Cut the zucchinis in half lengthwise, then cut them in half widthwise (if they are particularly long, cut them into thirds). Cut each half into 2 or 4 fry shapes depending on how wide your zucchinis are.
3. Beat the egg whites in a wide, shallow bowl. In another wide, shallow bowl, combine the breadcrumbs, herbs, if using, and salt and pepper to taste. Dip each zucchini fry into the whites then lightly into the breadcrumbs. Place the fries on the prepared baking sheet as you dip each one and bake for 15 to 20 minutes, flipping them halfway through, until browned and crisp.
4. Transfer to a bowl and serve immediately.

Sweet Potato Fries

SERVES 4

While ordering sweet potato fries at your burger joint upgrades your fry-eating experience (sweet potatoes are loaded with beta-carotene), if they're fried, they're still swimming in potentially unhealthy fats and loaded with calories. Bake your sweet potato fries and you'll trim calories by about a third, cut the fat in half, and completely eliminate the guilt. Cut your fries the same size for even baking, and don't overcrowd the pan so they stay crisp.

+ Extra-virgin olive oil cooking spray
+ 3 medium sweet potatoes
+ Salt

Step It Up!
Add seasonings such as paprika, garlic powder, onion powder, or chili powder.

1. Preheat the oven to 400°F.

2. Spray two baking sheets with cooking spray and place both sheets in the oven.

3. Scrub the sweet potatoes and cut each end to end into 8 wedges. Place them in a bowl, spray with cooking spray, and toss to coat well. Season with salt to taste and toss again.

4. One at a time, remove the baking sheets from the oven and place the sweet potatoes on the sheets cut side down.

5. Bake until the underside is crisp and lightly browned, 15 to 20 minutes. Remove the baking sheets from the oven and turn the sweet potatoes using a metal spatula. Bake until the second side is crisp and lightly browned, another 10 to 15 minutes. Remove from the sheet and serve immediately.

Doctor Mac and Cheese

SERVES 4 TO 6

Next time you get a craving for mac and cheese, grab this recipe. The difference between mine and the kind you find in a box: no fake cheese and lots of veggies (that will go unnoticed). Note that most orange cheddar is colored naturally by a seed called annatto, so as long as you're using real cheese your cheddar will likely be all natural, but check the label for artificial coloring just to be sure.

+ 12 ounces whole-wheat or other whole-grain pasta elbows or small shells
+ 1 (10-ounce) package frozen cauliflower florets, defrosted
+ 1 cup (2½ ounces) coarsely shredded cheddar cheese, plus 1/4 to 1/2 cup more for topping
+ 1 cup milk
+ 1/2 cup raw unsalted cashews, soaked in hot water to cover by 2 inches for at least 1 hour or overnight
+ 1 shallot, finely chopped
+ 2 garlic cloves, pressed through a garlic press
+ 1 tablespoon red wine vinegar, or to taste
+ 3/4 teaspoon sweet paprika
+ 1/4 teaspoon ground turmeric
+ 1/2 teaspoon salt, or to taste
+ 1/4 teaspoon freshly ground black pepper
+ 1/4 to 1/2 cup whole-wheat breadcrumbs

Continues ▸

1. Preheat the oven to 425°F.

2. Bring a large pot of water to a boil. Add the pasta and cook according to the package directions to al dente. Drain.

3. Meanwhile, make the sauce: In a blender or food processor, combine the cauliflower, cheese, milk, cashews, shallot, garlic, vinegar, paprika, turmeric, salt, and pepper and blend until smooth, scraping the sides of the machine as needed to get at everything. Add a little water if the mixture is too thick (you're looking for a fairly thick but still pourable consistency).

4. Place the pasta in a large bowl, add the sauce, and stir to combine. Transfer the pasta to a 9 by 9–inch baking pan and top with the bread-crumbs, followed by the remaining cheese. Place in the oven and bake for about 25 minutes, until browned on top and bubbly. Serve imme-diately.

Variation:

Gluten-Free Mac and Cheese: Use brown rice pasta and omit the breadcrumbs, or substitute toasted ground almonds or walnuts.

Eggplant Parmesan

SERVES 6 AS A SIDE

Eggplant is the star here, skipping the typical breading, frying, and loading up on cheese, for an eggplant Parm that leaves you light and satisfied. Tip: Freezing your mozzarella cheese for 30 minutes makes shredding easier and avoids cheese sticking to the grater. Omit the breadcrumbs to make the dish gluten-free.

+ Extra-virgin olive oil cooking spray
+ 2 large eggplants (about 2 pounds)
+ Salt and freshly ground black pepper
+ 1 recipe Simply Tomato Sauce (page 56) or low-sodium store-bought tomato sauce
+ 1 cup chopped fresh basil leaves, plus more for serving
+ 1/2 to 1 cup shredded fresh mozzarella cheese (2 to 4 ounces)
+ 1/4 to 1/2 cup grated Parmesan cheese
+ 1/4 cup whole-wheat breadcrumbs (optional)

1. Preheat the oven to 450°F. Spray two baking sheets with cooking spray.
2. Peel each eggplant if you like or leave them unpeeled and slice them about 1/2-inch thick. Place the slices on the baking sheets in a single layer. Lightly spray the tops of the slices with cooking spray and season each slice with salt and pepper to taste. Place in the oven and

Continues ▶

bake until deeply browned on top and a fork inserted into a slice goes in easily, about 30 minutes. Remove the eggplants from the oven. Remove the slices from the baking sheets and transfer them to a plate to cool. Lower the oven temperature to 350°F.

3. Spray an 8 by 12–inch baking pan with about 1 cup of the tomato sauce. Cover with half of the eggplant slices, followed by another cup of tomato sauce. Sprinkle on half of the basil, followed by half of the mozzarella cheese and half of the Parmesan cheese. Add a second and final layer of eggplant and repeat with the remaining tomato sauce, basil, and mozzarella and Parmesan cheeses. If using the breadcrumbs, sprinkle them over the top of the dish, then add a grinding of pepper.

4. Place in the oven and bake uncovered until the cheese is melted, the tops are lightly browned, and the dish is sizzling hot, about 30 minutes. Cut into squares and serve.

Super-Crisp Chicken Wings

SERVES 4 TO 6

These wings are the stay-fit option to fatty bar food, as they are equally crisp and every bit as tasty as their deep-fried counterparts. If perhaps you and your family have been extra-active today, consider adding 2 tablespoons butter to the hot sauce mixture for a little extra richness.

Wings

- 2½ pounds chicken wings, tips removed, drumettes and flats separated
- 2 teaspoons baking powder
- 1½ teaspoons salt
- 1 teaspoon garlic powder
- 1 teaspoon onion powder
- 1/4 cup hot sauce
- 1 tablespoon fresh lime juice

Dipping sauce

- 1 cup plain Greek yogurt
- 1 tablespoon minced fresh mint
- 1 teaspoon freshly grated lemon zest
- 2 teaspoons fresh lemon juice
- 1/4 teaspoon salt
- Celery sticks

Continues ▶

1. To make the wings: Line a baking sheet with aluminum foil and set a wire rack on top of it. (Make sure your rack isn't the kind with plastic feet!)

2. Pat the wings dry with paper towels. Place the wings in a large bowl, sprinkle with the baking powder, salt, garlic powder, and onion powder, and toss until evenly coated (putting on a disposable glove and massaging it in with your hand is a good way of accomplishing this). Place the wings on the rack, leaving a little space between each, and leave on the counter for 30 minutes.

3. While the wings are resting, preheat the oven to 450°F.

4. Place the wings in the oven and roast for 20 minutes. Using tongs, flip the wings and roast until very crisp and well browned, about 25 minutes longer.

5. While the wings are roasting, make the yogurt dipping sauce: In a medium bowl, whisk together all the ingredients.

6. Transfer the wings to a heatproof bowl, add the hot sauce and lime juice, toss to thoroughly coat, and serve with the dipping sauce and celery sticks.

MAKE IT A MEAL 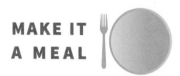 Serve with a crisp green salad and Garlicky Butternut Squash Mash (page 106).

 Time-saver: Cut the wings into drumettes and flats up to a day ahead. If you have a bit of fridge space, after tossing the wings with the seasonings, set the wings on the wire racks atop the baking sheets and place in the refrigerator uncovered for up to 24 hours. Remove them when you go to preheat the oven. As a bonus, they will be even crispier when they come to the table.

Oven-Fried Chicken

SERVES 4

A quick coating of buttermilk, a toss with oats and flour, and a turn in the oven makes for chicken that's crisp on the outside, tender on the inside, just like classic fried chicken. Keeping the skin on the chicken provides extra "glue" for the crispy coating, but if you're watching your calories, you can remove the skin. To further cut calories, choose breasts rather than drumsticks.

+ Extra-virgin olive oil cooking spray
+ 2½ pounds bone-in chicken drumsticks or breasts, skin kept on or removed
+ 1½ cups quick-cooking rolled oats
+ 1/4 cup whole-wheat flour
+ 1 teaspoon garlic powder
+ 1 teaspoon onion powder
+ 1 teaspoon dried thyme
+ 2½ teaspoons salt
+ 1/4 teaspoon freshly ground black pepper
+ 1/2 cup buttermilk

1. Preheat the oven to 425°F. Line a baking sheet with foil and set a wire rack atop it. Spray the rack with cooking spray.

2. In a zip-top bag, combine the rolled oats, flour, garlic powder, onion powder, thyme, 2 teaspoons of the salt, and the pepper.

Continues ▶

Fear of Frying

An occasional indulgence aside, deep-fried fast food is best avoided entirely. Some oils are much better to cook with than others, but frying any oil inevitably breaks it down, turning the molecules rancid and creating chemicals that may even be carcinogenic—enough to put the fear of frying in you. Overcooking can also destroy certain vitamins and degrade enzymes and phytochemicals. There are different levels of cooking that require less oil, lower heat, and shorter cooking times that you can experiment with, or try drizzling raw extra-virgin olive oil over a simple dish of poached fish (page 145) or steamed greens (page 102) after they're cooked to enjoy the unadulterated benefits of the fat.

3. Pat the chicken dry with paper towels. Place the chicken in a shallow baking pan and pour the buttermilk over it. Sprinkle in the remaining 1/2 teaspoon of salt and toss, turning to coat all sides of the chicken. Remove the chicken pieces one at a time from the buttermilk, allowing excess to drip off. Place the chicken pieces one at a time in the oat mixture and shake to coat well.

4. Place the chicken pieces on the prepared rack, leaving space between each, and spray with cooking spray. Place in the oven and bake for about 45 minutes, turning once halfway through and giving another spray of cooking spray (make sure to remove the pan from the oven before spraying), until the chicken is browned and the juices run clear. If you have an instant-read thermometer, the chicken is done when it reads 165°F.

5. Remove from the oven and serve immediately.

Step It Up!
Marinate the chicken overnight before baking. Increase the buttermilk to 1½ cups and add 2 garlic cloves, pressed through a garlic press. Keep the chicken in the pan, cover, and refrigerate from between 5 and 12 hours.

Spaghetti and Meatballs

SERVES 4

These kid-tested meatballs skip the breadcrumbs and cheese typically added to the mix while keeping their comfort food appeal. Since the meatballs contain no fillers, there's nothing standing between you and the meat, making them a highly satisfying dinner choice and ideal for those who are gluten-free. You'll save your carbs for whole-grain spaghetti to complete the classic combination, or go lighter by choosing Nudels (page 109) or spaghetti squash (page 110)—and get in an extra serving of nutrient-dense veggies while you're at it!

+ 1 pound lean ground turkey, pork, beef, or a combination of pork and beef
+ 1 teaspoon dried oregano
+ 1½ teaspoons Italian seasoning
+ 1½ teaspoons garlic powder
+ 1½ teaspoons onion powder
+ 1 teaspoon salt
+ 1/4 teaspoon freshly ground black pepper
+ 1 recipe Simply Tomato Sauce (page 56) or low-sodium store-bought tomato sauce

Pasta options:

+ Brown rice spaghetti or other whole-grain pasta
+ Nudels (page 109) or cooked spaghetti squash (page 110)

Continues ▶

1. In a large bowl, combine the ground meat, oregano, Italian seasoning, garlic powder, onion powder, salt, and pepper; wearing a disposable glove or using your clean hands, mix very well to incorporate all the ingredients. Form the mixture into about 16 equal-size balls measuring about 1½ inches each. Place on a baking sheet or a couple of large plates.

2. Just after you've brought your tomato sauce to a simmer (you don't need to cook it before adding the meatballs), gently add the meatballs using a slotted spoon and lightly stir to coat the meatballs in the sauce. Bring back to a simmer, then reduce the heat to low, cover, and simmer for 30 minutes, or until the meatballs are cooked through.

3. Serve over the noodles of your choice.

Snacks

Snacking is important—if done correctly it can actually help to keep the weight off. These are some of my favorite make-ahead snacks, little protein- or veggie-packed bites to get me through to the next meal without breaking the calorie bank. The Chickpea Crunch (page 205) doubles as a vegetarian protein side, the Crispy Kale Chips (page 206) are a gold mine of greens to be devoured, and Power Bites (page 212) are the freshest-tasting energy bar you'll ever eat. I've also included a healthy chip recipe (page 208) and two nut and seed mixes (pages 209 to 210); if you don't have the time to make your own, there are many quality brands for you to choose from. Go for those made with olive oil or another quality oil and that are low in sodium.

Grab and Go Snack Options

❖ Handful of nuts or seeds, such as almonds, walnuts, peanuts, pecans, pistachios, pumpkin seeds, or sunflower seeds

❖ 1 cup plain Greek yogurt with fruit or a drizzle of honey (or any of the yogurt breakfast bowl options on page 18)

❖ Chunk (about 1 ounce) of cheese, such as cheddar, mozzarella, or Swiss

❖ 1/2 cup cottage cheese or ricotta with a drizzle of honey

❖ Hummus (page 44), guacamole (page 59), or salsa (pages 50 to 54) with vegetable sticks or spooned into endive leaves

❖ Slice of whole-grain toast or whole-grain English muffin with 1/2 tablespoon all-natural, no-sugar-added nut butter

❖ Mini pizza: half of a whole-grain English muffin toasted with tomato sauce (page 56) and shredded mozzarella cheese

❖ Apple slices with about 2 teaspoons peanut butter or almond butter

❖ Tortilla warmed in the microwave and spread with a dip (pages 41 to 60)

❖ Edamame (fresh soybeans in the shell) drizzled with olive oil and a pinch of salt

❖ Sliced tomato with a sprinkle of feta cheese

❖ Hard-boiled egg

❖ Piece of dark chocolate (minimum 70% cocoa) with almond butter

For more snack ideas, check out the many options in *The Doctor's Diet*.

Chickpea Crunch

MAKES ABOUT 2 CUPS

When chickpeas are roasted they become crisp and crunchy—a perfect finger food and a lower-calorie alternative to nuts. And they do double duty as a side or salad topper. The recipe is easily scaled up for entertaining.

+ 2 (15-ounce) cans no-salt-added chickpeas, rinsed and drained, or 3 cups cooked dried chickpeas
+ 1 tablespoon extra-virgin olive oil
+ 1 teaspoon garlic powder
+ 1 teaspoon dried rosemary, oregano, thyme, or other spice
+ 1/2 teaspoon salt, or to taste
+ 1/4 teaspoon freshly ground black pepper

1. Preheat the oven to 400°F.
2. Pat the chickpeas dry with paper towels (make sure to dry them thoroughly for crispiest results).
3. In a large bowl, combine the oil, garlic powder, rosemary, salt, and pepper and stir to combine. Add the chickpeas and toss to thoroughly coat.
4. Spread the chickpeas evenly over a baking sheet and bake for about 30 minutes, until lightly browned and crisp. Pour into a bowl and serve.

 Make Ahead: Canned chickpeas are a great time-saver, but using dried chickpeas will save you money. If you have the time to cook up a big pot of chickpeas, cool them and put 1½ cup portions (a 15-ounce can is 1½ cups) into zip-top freezer bags. Freeze and thaw as needed.

Crispy Kale Chips

MAKES A NICE, BIG BOWLFUL

Kale chips are a happy surprise to many people who've never heard of or tried them; like ordinary potato chips, it's also very hard to stop at just a few!

The key to crispy kale chips every time is making sure you dry them thoroughly (so they bake rather than steam) and baking low and slow—at 250°F for up to 40 minutes—so your chips are evenly crisp throughout. This is a simple recipe, but note that it does require some time commitment.

Crispy kale chips will keep for two to three months in an airtight container. So if you've got a plot of kale growing in your garden or kale is on sale at the market, why not dedicate a couple hours to kale chip making?

+ 2 bunches kale (any type)
+ Extra-virgin olive oil cooking spray
+ 1/4 to 1/2 teaspoon salt
+ Sprinkle of herbs of your choice, such as garlic powder, onion powder, chili powder, or Italian spices (optional)

1. Preheat the oven to 250°F.
2. Remove the stems from the kale and tear the leaves into bite-size pieces. Wash and thoroughly dry the kale.
3. Place the kale in a large bowl. Spray with cooking spray and add the salt and herbs, if using (you may need to do this in two batches). Massage the oil and seasonings onto each kale piece to evenly distribute the oil.

4. Spread the kale out onto two 9 by 13–inch baking sheets (you may need to do this in two batches). Bake the kale until the leaves look crisp with no wet spots and they crumble when rubbed between your fingers, 30 to 40 minutes.

5. Remove from the oven and cool to room temperature. Pour into a bowl and serve.

Sweet Potato Chips

SERVES 4

If you can fry it, there's a good chance you can roast it too, with equally tasty and healthier results. Make sure to keep your sweet potato slices uniform so they bake evenly with no burnt edges. If you happen to have a mandoline slicer, this recipe is your chance to take it out of the box and use it.

+ Extra-virgin olive oil cooking spray
+ 1 medium sweet potato, scrubbed but not peeled and sliced 1/8-inch thick
+ Salt

1. Preheat the oven to 400°F. Spray a baking sheet with cooking spray.
2. Lay the sweet potato slices on the prepared sheet in a single layer, spray the tops with cooking spray, and sprinkle with salt to taste. Place in the oven and bake for 20 to 25 minutes, turning them once halfway through, until the chips are browned and crisp.
3. Remove from the oven, pour into a bowl, and serve.

Toasted Nuts 101

MAKES 2 CUPS

Why toast your own nuts when you can simply open a bag and dig in? See below for five good reasons. If you don't have the time to toast your own, go for low-salt packaged nuts made without hydrogenated oils. The recipe easily scales up; make enough to fill a couple of baking sheets so you'll have plenty for snack packs to toss into lunchboxes or take on the road.

+ 2 cups raw unsalted almonds, cashews, pecans, walnuts, pistachios, or a mixture
+ 2 teaspoons to 1 tablespoon extra-virgin olive oil (optional)
+ 1/4 teaspoon salt, or to taste (optional; if using oil)
+ Sprinkle of herbs or spices (optional; if using oil)

1. Preheat the oven to 350°F.
2. In a medium bowl, toss the nuts with the oil, if using. Add the salt, if using, and herbs, if using, and toss again.
3. Place in the oven and roast for 5 minutes, then stir and roast for another 5 to 10 minutes, until lightly browned and aromatic.
4. Remove from the oven and transfer to a plate to cool. Store in an airtight container for up to a month, or fill snack bags with 1/4-cup portions to toss into lunchboxes.

 Time-saver: Toast the nuts in a skillet on the stovetop over medium heat, stirring often, until evenly browned and aromatic, about 5 minutes. Transfer to a plate to cool.

Chili-Toasted Pumpkin Seeds

MAKES 1 CUP

These little seeds make a tasty quick snack and are endlessly adaptable to whatever herbs or spices you wish to add. Pumpkin seeds are rich in protein and minerals, including iron, magnesium, manganese, phosphorus, and zinc, and a valuable source of omega-3 fatty acids—enjoy them often! Note that chili powder is a spice blend (as opposed to chile powder, made from ground chiles); favor chili powder with no added salt.

To roast your pumpkin seeds in the oven (a good option for making larger batches), spread them out on a baking sheet and bake in a preheated 350°F oven for 10 to 12 minutes, stirring once, until lightly browned and fragrant.

+ 1 cup pumpkin seeds
+ 1 teaspoon extra-virgin olive oil
+ 1 teaspoon no-salt-added chili powder
+ 1/8 to 1/4 teaspoon salt

1. In a medium bowl, toss together the pumpkin seeds, oil, chili powder, and salt.
2. Heat a medium skillet over medium heat and add the pumpkin seeds. Cook, stirring constantly, until the pumpkin seeds are lightly browned and fragrant, about 5 minutes.
3. Remove from the heat and pour in a bowl to cool. They will keep, stored in a lidded jar, for up to a month.

Why Roast at Home?

1. Your nuts will be hot-out-of-the-oven fresh.
2. They'll be lower in sodium (you choose how much goes in them).
3. They'll be lighter, made with good-quality oils (skip the oil for dry-roasted nuts).
4. They'll be lighter on your wallet.
5. It's almost no work at all.

The Skinny on Nuts

What if I told you there was a pill with few or no side effects, and if you took it three or four times a week it might help to keep your weight down and decrease your risk of heart disease and might even help you live longer? You'd do it, right? Well, I'm actually referring to eating nuts! While nuts aren't a low-calorie food per se, eating them as part of a balanced diet (a serving is generally no more than a handful) may actually help you lose weight. The likely reason: nuts are loaded with protein and healthy fats to fill you up; they'll keep you satisfied so you won't feel hungry later, making mindless snacking between meals unlikely.

Variations:

Curry Toasted Pumpkin Seeds: Substitute 1 teaspoon curry powder (your choice of mild, medium, or hot) for the chili powder.

Spicy Toasted Pumpkin Seeds: Substitute 1/4 to 1/2 teaspoon ground cayenne for the chili powder.

Spicy Smoky Toasted Pumpkin Seeds: Substitute 1/4 to 1/2 teaspoon ground chipotle for the chili powder.

Garlic and Onion Toasted Pumpkin Seeds: Substitute 1/4 teaspoon garlic powder and 1/4 teaspoon onion powder for the chili powder.

Power Bites

MAKES 32 SMALLER 1-INCH BITES OR 16 LARGER-SIZE BARS

Tangy, nutty bursts of energy, these no-bake bites are lighter and lower in sugar than store-bought energy bars. The flavor, reminiscent of PB&J, will make you smile like a kid. Feel free to play around with different combinations of fruits, nuts, and seeds; some ideas to get you started include mini dark chocolate chips, shredded coconut, hemp seeds, and dried blueberries.

+ 2 tablespoons virgin coconut oil, plus more for the pan
+ 1 cup raw unsalted almonds
+ 1/2 cup raw unsalted sunflower seeds
+ 1/2 cup raw unsalted hulled pumpkin seeds
+ 2 teaspoons chia seeds
+ 2 teaspoons sesame seeds
+ 1 cup dried unsulfured apricots, chopped
+ 1/2 cup dried dates, pitted and chopped
+ 1/2 cup raisins
+ 2 tablespoons all-natural no-sugar-added almond butter
+ 2 tablespoons honey
+ 2 teaspoons fresh lemon juice
+ 2 teaspoons pure vanilla extract
+ 1/2 teaspoon salt

1. Lightly oil an 8 by 8–inch pan with coconut oil and set aside.
2. Place the almonds in a food processor and pulse until they are medium chopped. Add the sunflower seeds, pumpkin seeds, chia

Energy Bars—or Candy Bars?

While there are some balanced-nutrition energy bars out there, many have a high sugar content, whether it's refined sugar or a more wholesome sweetener. A good few are based on soy protein isolate, a refined form of soy that can be hard to digest; skip these and favor back-to-nature types featuring nuts and dried fruits. Choose bars in the 200 calorie range and watch the carb count (some bars contain more than 40 grams of carbohydrates!), or play it safe by sharing a bar with your workout partner.

seeds, and sesame seeds and pulse a few more times, just until the nuts and seeds are well mixed (don't overprocess or you may wind up with nut butter). Transfer the mixture to a bowl and set aside.

3. Add the apricots, dates, raisins, almond butter, honey, coconut oil, lemon juice, vanilla, and salt to the food processor (no need to wash it out first) and process into a paste with small chunks still intact.

4. Add the nut-seed mixture and pulse until the ingredients are well distributed and combined. The texture will form a sticky mass (it shouldn't be loose). Lightly dampen your hands with water, scoop out the mixture, and evenly press it into the prepared pan, smoothing the top.

5. Place the bars into the refrigerator for 1 hour or the freezer for 30 minutes to set, then slice them into 1-inch bites or larger-size bars if you prefer. Store the power bites in an airtight container.

 Make Ahead: These bars keep well—unrefrigerated they will be fresh for up to 2 weeks, refrigerated for up to 1 month—so make a batch or two to have them handy to bring on a hike, pass around at a meeting, or tuck into a lunchbox.

Go Seeds!

Seeds are not only unique and diverse in their varying tastes, textures, and uses, but they are all superfoods. Chia and flax have been in the limelight as of late (see the sidebars on pages 23 and 25), but don't forget sunflower, pumpkin, and sesame seeds! They are all great sources of protein and are high in fiber, heart-healthy monounsaturated fats, vitamin E, and minerals, especially zinc.

Sunflower seeds promote healthy digestion and are rich in folate (again, that's folic acid), which is particularly important for women during pregnancy and may help reduce high blood pressure. The phenomenal pumpkin seed is loaded with omega-3 fatty acids and antioxidants that enhance immune activity. Sesame seeds are high in calcium, contain cholesterol-fighting fibers, and may help prevent high blood pressure.

Enjoy your seeds in your desserts, sprinkle them on salads, toss them into chicken or tuna salad, or simply pop a few into your mouth for a wonderfully snappy snack.

Sweet Treats

Diets inevitably fail when they are too rigid. At the other extreme, the average American eats 20-plus teaspoons of added sugar a day, and two out of three of us are overweight or obese. In *The Doctor's Diet* STAT Plan, we broke up with sugar, but if you've gotten back down to a healthy weight, now you can enjoy the occasional sweet treat.

There's nothing wrong with dessert, if you're careful. In fact, we are hardwired to like sweet foods: way back during hunter-gatherer times, sweet taste was one of the ways we could recognize a food as safe to eat. What's more, sweet is tied to the reward centers in our brains, and a little can help relieve stress, pain, and minor depression. The trick is to know when to stop. Favor desserts containing protein, whole grains, and unrefined sweeteners such as honey and pure maple syrup, as these ingredients help to slow down the absorption of sugar and leave you feeling satisfied rather than ready to reach for the bottom of the cookie jar.

Don't blow your health budget on dessert, and eat your dessert *as* dessert. You don't want to wake up and eat banana pudding for breakfast, go on to crispy rice treats for lunch, munch on a brownie for an afternoon snack, and dine on ice cream for dinner . . . you get the picture. Moderation and mindfulness is key. Now it's time to enjoy your sweets more than you've ever enjoyed them before!

Peaches and Cream

SERVES 2

Dessert doesn't have to be an elaborate affair. A little something sweet, a simple serving of fruit for example, is often all that's called for to complete a meal. For a special treat, substitute all-natural frozen yogurt or ice cream for the yogurt.

+ 1 peach
+ Squeeze of lemon juice
+ 3 tablespoons plain Greek yogurt
+ 1 tablespoon honey
+ Ground nutmeg (optional)

Step It Up!
Strain the yogurt through a strainer lined with a paper towel for an hour or two to thicken it into yogurt "cream."

Cut the peach in half and remove the pit. Extend the hole where the pit was to make enough room to fit the yogurt. Squeeze a little lemon juice over the peach halves, top with yogurt, and drizzle with honey. Dust with nutmeg, if using.

Variation:

Grilled Peaches with Greek Yogurt: Spray the cut sides of the peach halves with cooking spray and place cut side down on a grill or grill pan preheated to medium-high heat. Cook until slightly charred but retaining their shape, about 2 minutes per side, then proceed with the recipe as above. If your peaches are really juicy and become too soft to stuff, quarter the peach halves, toss with lemon juice and honey, spoon into bowls, and top with the yogurt.

Sliced Apples with Honey

SERVES 1

Simpler than pie! Choose any variety of apple you like, from McIntosh to good old Granny Smith. Feel free to swap in pears when they're in season.

+ 1 crisp apple, cored and sliced into wedges
+ 1 tablespoon honey
+ Handful of slivered almonds
+ Large pinch of ground cinnamon

Arrange the apple wedges on a plate, drizzle with the honey, and top with the almonds and cinnamon. Serve immediately.

Super Almonds!

Almonds are considered a superfood because of their heart-healthy nutritional benefits. Almonds have an impressive profile, including powerful antioxidants, anti-inflammatories, healthy fats, fiber, vitamin E, and potassium, calcium, and other minerals. On top of all that goodness, their sweet flavor and toothsome texture makes almonds taste wonderful. A handful of raw or roasted almonds (see page 209 for how to roast almonds) makes for a convenient and super-healthy snack.

Dark Chocolate Mousse

SERVES 4

Skeptical? One bite of this velvety rich avocado-based mousse will make you an avocado-for-dessert believer. Turn to page 67 to learn about the benefits of avocados.

+ 2 medium ripe avocados, cut in half, pit removed, and flesh scooped out
+ 1/2 cup unsweetened cocoa powder
+ 1/3 cup honey or pure maple syrup, or to taste
+ 1/2 cup almond milk, another nut milk, or dairy milk
+ 1 tablespoon fresh lemon juice
+ 1/2 teaspoon vanilla extract

1. In a food processor, combine all the ingredients and process until silky smooth and creamy, 3 to 4 minutes (don't skimp on the time), scraping the sides of the machine once or twice, as needed.
2. Spoon into bowls, cover, and refrigerate until cold before serving. The mousse will keep, covered and refrigerated, for up to 3 days.

Chocolate: The "Sinful" Antioxidant

By now most of us have heard that real chocolate is considered healthy (some of the best news ever!), but let's get some things clear before we go too cuckoo for cocoa.

Chocolate is derived from the seeds and pods of the cacao tree, predominantly grown in Central and South America and in West Africa. Raw cacao contains one of the most impressive arsenals of antioxidant compounds seen in nature's edible cornucopia. On top of that, cacao is an exceptional source of minerals, particularly iron, magnesium, phosphorus, zinc, potassium, and even calcium and selenium. It also has some B vitamins, notably a fair amount of riboflavin. All of these nutrients combined makes for a very nourishing food with real therapeutic action, as is supported by study after study.

However, no doctor is about to prescribe candy bars anytime soon. Much of the chocolate used in your typical candy bar is highly refined and mixed with artificial ingredients and a ton of sugar. For maximum health benefits, look for simple dark chocolate that is at least 70% cocoa and eat in moderation (about half an ounce at a time). I eat a small square of dark chocolate almost every day, and for a satisfying snack, I'll go up to 88 percent dark chocolate and dip it in some almond butter.

Light and Airy Mousse with Cherries

SERVES 2 TO 3

This lightly sweetened mousse interpretation is elegant yet super-simple to put together and an excellent ending to any meal.

+ 1 cup frozen unsweetened cherries
+ 1/4 teaspoon pure vanilla extract
+ Pinch of ground allspice
+ Pinch of ground nutmeg
+ 1 cup ricotta cheese
+ 1 tablespoon unsweetened cocoa powder
+ 2 tablespoons honey
+ 2 teaspoons mini dark chocolate chips (optional)

1. Place the cherries in a bowl and set aside for an hour or so to defrost them (or defrost them in the refrigerator overnight).
2. Add the vanilla, allspice, and nutmeg and lightly mash the cherries to bring out their juices and combine the ingredients.
3. Place the ricotta in a medium bowl. Add the cocoa powder and whisk it in to incorporate it, then whisk in the honey.
4. Divide the ricotta between two bowls or parfait glasses, top with the cherries and their juices, and serve, with the chocolate chips sprinkled on top, if using.

Banana Pudding

SERVES 4

Chia seeds are the secret ingredient that makes this pudding creamy (see page 23 to learn about their amazing powers), and potassium- rich bananas are blended right in for added richness and flavor. Skip the yogurt if you're dairy sensitive, and look for white chia seeds rather than black if you'd like a lighter colored pudding.

+ 2 ripe bananas
+ 1 cup unsweetened coconut milk (not cream of coconut)
+ 1 tablespoon pure maple syrup or honey
+ 1 teaspoon pure vanilla extract
+ 1/4 teaspoon ground cardamom
+ 1/4 cup chia seeds
+ 2 broken-up all-natural graham crackers or a handful of toasted chopped almonds
+ 1/4 cup whisked plain Greek yogurt (optional)

1. In a blender, combine the bananas, coconut milk, maple syrup, vanilla, and cardamom and process until smooth. Add the chia seeds and blend until completely combined.

2. Pour into a container or individual serving bowls, cover, and refrigerate for 30 minutes to 1 hour for the chia seeds to plump up.

3. Serve, with the graham crackers stirred into the pudding and topped with Greek yogurt, if using.

Peanut Butter Bliss

MAKES ABOUT 2 DOZEN

Most days a square of dark chocolate dipped into the peanut butter jar is all I need to satisfy my sweet tooth. These little rounds expand on the concept, adding fiber-rich flaxseed and whole oats for extra fuel.

+ 2/3 cup quick-cooking oats
+ 1/2 cup unsweetened toasted dried coconut
+ 1/2 cup ground flaxseed
+ 1/3 cup mini dark chocolate chips
+ 1/2 cup smooth all-natural no-sugar-added peanut butter
+ 1/3 cup honey or pure maple syrup

1. In a large bowl, combine the oats, coconut, flaxseed, and chocolate chips. Add the peanut butter and honey and mix together with your hands until the ingredients are well incorporated.
2. Wash your hands to clear them of sticky dough, then roll the mixture into 1-inch balls. Place in a storage container and store in the refrigerator, where they will keep ready to eat for up to 2 weeks, or in the freezer, where they will keep for up to 2 months.

Honey and Maple Syrup: A Little Goes a Long Way

Recent research indicates that people whose diets are highest in refined sugar are the most at risk for heart disease. But our brains are hardwired to be attracted to the taste of sweet, so I'd never ask you to give up sweets completely. What I *am* asking you to do is to consider natural sweeteners—honey and maple syrup are my favorites—when you've got a hankering for a little something sweet. And let *little* be your guideline, as a small amount of a quality sweetener goes a long way. Once you've broken the sugar habit, you'll find yourself satisfied with less of it and enjoy just a drizzle of honey atop your yogurt or a small serving of a dessert sweetened with pure maple syrup.

Honey contains natural antioxidants, enzymes, amino acids, vitamins, and minerals, and humans have been enjoying this nectar of the gods for at least 10,000 years. Honey is not low in sugar, but it is lower on the glycemic index, meaning its sugar is more slowly absorbed into the bloodstream rather than producing the shock and crash that's associated with refined sugar. When you purchase honey that's labeled *raw*, you're assured that all of its nutrients are intact.

Maple syrup is produced by boiling down the sap of the maple tree; it is high in minerals, particularly manganese and zinc, and B vitamins. Maple syrup is filled with antioxidants, and like honey, its sugar is more gradually absorbed into the bloodstream than refined sugar. Make sure to read your maple syrup label and look for *pure* maple syrup.

Another sweetener worth seeking out is molasses; this sweet, dark, and sticky liquid is what's left over from the sugar-making process and contains impressive amounts of calcium, magnesium, potassium, and iron. Blackstrap molasses is the most nutritious variety; it has a very strong flavor so is best used in small amounts. Note that most brown sugar (unless it is labeled *unrefined*) is simply refined white sugar with a token amount of molasses added back in for color, often with the assistance of food colorings.

Crispy Rice Treats

MAKES 16 FULL-SIZE TREATS OR 25 BITE-SIZE TREATS

This favorite comfort food just got a makeover by swapping in whole-grain crispies, and the glue that holds them together is peanut butter and honey rather than marshmallows heavy in high-fructose corn syrup. With complex carbs from the brown rice cereal and healthy fats and protein from the peanut butter, these go beyond the typical treat territory and can even be enjoyed as an alternative to energy bars.

+ Light olive oil or coconut oil cooking spray
+ 3 cups crispy brown rice cereal
+ 2/3 cup light honey or brown rice syrup
+ 1/2 cup smooth all-natural no-sugar-added peanut butter
+ 6 ounces (1 cup) dark chocolate chips (optional)

1. Line an 8 by 8–inch baking dish with aluminum foil so that it extends up the sides and over the edges of the pan. Spray the foil generously with cooking spray. Spray a rubber spatula with cooking spray as well.

2. Pour the brown rice cereal into a bowl and have it ready.

3. In a small saucepan, combine the honey and peanut butter and heat, stirring often, until the peanut butter melts into the honey, about 3 minutes. Remove from the heat.

4. Immediately pour the peanut butter mixture over the rice cereal and quickly and thoroughly mix it in with the prepared spatula. Pour the mixture into the prepared pan and push it down evenly with the spatula. If you're not including the chocolate layer, cool, then lift the treats

from the pan using the extended foil edges and place on a cutting board. Slide the foil out from under the treats and cut the treats into squares.

5. If making a chocolate layer, place the pan in the refrigerator while you melt the chocolate. Place the chocolate chips in a microwave-safe bowl and melt the chocolate in the microwave for 30-second intervals, stirring in between, until the chocolate is fully melted (be careful not to over-microwave, or the chocolate may burn).

6. Quickly pour the melted chocolate over the rice cereal mixture and spread it evenly with a rubber spatula. Place in the freezer for about 1 hour to firm up, then lift the treats from the pan using the extended foil edges and place on a cutting board. Slide the foil out from under the treats and cut the treats into squares.

7. Store in the refrigerator for up to 5 days, or individually wrap the squares and keep them in the freezer until you're ready to thaw and eat them.

Nuts for Brownies

MAKES 16 FULL-SIZE BROWNIES OR 25 BROWNIE BITES

Everyone needs a chocolate treat once in a while, myself included! Brownies are one of my favorite guilty pleasures, but with these you can lose the guilt (as long as you stick to just one!). The nut butter base makes them incredibly moist and fudgy (and notice that there's no flour used here—it would only get in the way of their extreme fudginess), and you get a bonus protein boost that fills you up and keeps you going midday (which is exactly the opposite of what the typical refined sugar and flour brownies do to you—quick high, soon followed by a nose-dive crash).

Note that because these brownies are so moist, they can be a bit crumbly when cutting; try wiping your knife between cuts as you slice them, or freeze the pan of brownies for a half hour before cutting.

+ Light olive oil or coconut oil cooking spray
+ 1 cup creamy all-natural no-sugar-added almond or cashew butter
+ 2 large eggs
+ 1/2 cup pure maple syrup or honey
+ 1 teaspoon pure vanilla extract
+ 1/2 teaspoon pure almond extract
+ 1/3 cup unsweetened cocoa powder
+ 1/2 teaspoon baking soda
+ 1/4 teaspoon salt
+ 1/3 cup dark chocolate chips

1. Position an oven rack at the middle position and preheat the oven to 350°F. Line an 8 by 8–inch baking dish with aluminum foil so that it extends up the sides and over the edges of the pan. Spray the foil generously with cooking spray.

2. In a large bowl, vigorously whisk the almond butter with a fork until smooth (if it is overly stiff, add a small amount of water to smooth it out). Add the eggs, maple syrup, and vanilla and almond extracts and beat with a whisk until combined.

3. In a separate bowl, whisk together the cocoa powder, baking soda, and salt. Slowly add the dry ingredients to the almond butter mixture, beating until smooth. Fold in the chocolate chips. Evenly pour the batter into the prepared pan, place in the oven, and bake until set in the center and a toothpick inserted in the center comes out mostly clean with a few crumbs, 20 to 25 minutes.

4. Place the pan on a wire rack to cool completely, about 1 hour. Lift the brownies from the pan using the extended foil edges and place on a cutting board. Slide the foil out from under the brownies and cut the brownies into squares. The brownies can be stored in an airtight container in the refrigerator for up to a week or frozen for several months.

Raspberry Almond Thumbprint Cookies

MAKES 20 COOKIES

These cookies are quick, foolproof, and an absolute treat. Using almond flour instead of wheat flour boosts their protein content, adds moistness, and results in a gluten-free cookie. This recipe requires both turning on your oven and using an electric mixer, but if your kitchen is equipped with both, I urge you to give it a try, as the results make it well worth the additional effort.

Almond flour is made from finely ground blanched almonds; it is high in protein and low in carbohydrates and sugars. It can be found in the gluten-free section of supermarkets and natural food stores. Feel free to fill the centers with a low-sugar favorite jam, making sure to avoid jams loaded with high-fructose corn syrup and other artificial sweeteners. Enjoying cookies made with almond flour and sweetened with healthier jam means you're less likely to have a spike in blood sugar after snacking, avoiding the sugar crash many of us get from eating super-sweet cookies.

+ 1/4 cup finely chopped raw unsalted almonds
+ 2 cups almond flour
+ 1 teaspoon baking powder
+ 1/4 teaspoon salt
+ 1/3 cup virgin coconut oil
+ 1/2 cup honey
+ 1/2 teaspoon pure almond extract
+ 1/2 teaspoon pure vanilla extract
+ 1 egg
+ About 1/4 cup low-sugar raspberry jam

1. Preheat the oven to 350°F. Line two 12 by 17–inch baking sheets with parchment paper.

2. Place the chopped almonds in a small bowl.

3. Sift the almond flour, baking powder, and salt into a medium bowl and set aside.

4. In the bowl of an electric mixer fitted with the paddle attachment, cream the coconut oil and honey until smooth, about 1 minute. Add the almond and vanilla extracts and beat to combine. On medium speed, add the egg and beat until the mixture appears homogenous, about 1 minute. Using a rubber spatula, scrape the insides of the bowl and beat for another 30 seconds. Turn off the mixer, add the dry ingredients, and mix the dough until it forms a loose mass. The dough will be a bit crumbly but will hold together when squeezed.

5. Divide the dough into 20 equal pieces. You may do this by using a small ice cream scoop or by rolling the dough into a log and slicing into portions. Roll each piece into a ball and then roll each ball into the chopped almonds, pressing so the almonds stick to the dough. Place the cookies on the baking sheets, leaving about 1½ inches of space between each. Using your thumbs, press a small, deep indentation into the center of each cookie. Fill each cookie with about 1/2 teaspoon of jam.

6. Place in the oven and bake for 10 minutes, or until the edges of the cookies are golden brown. Remove the cookies from the oven and place on wire racks to cool completely.

Frozen Lime Cheesecake Bites

MAKES 16 FULL-SIZE CHEESECAKE BARS OR 25 CHEESECAKE BITES

Here's something new for you: cheesecake made from cashews! You won't miss the cream cheese, as cashews become amazingly creamy when blended, making this dessert perfect for the dairy-free and vegans among us. The bonus is a substantial dose of protein and heart-protective fats with every cashew-packed bite.

+ Light olive oil or coconut oil cooking spray

Crust

+ 12 all-natural graham crackers, broken into pieces
+ 3 tablespoons melted virgin coconut oil

Filling

+ 2 cups raw cashews, soaked in hot water to cover for at least 4 hours or overnight and drained
+ 1/2 cup unsweetened coconut milk (not cream of coconut)
+ 1/2 cup fresh lime juice
+ 1/3 cup light-colored honey or maple syrup
+ 3 tablespoons virgin coconut oil, melted
+ 2 tablespoons grated lime zest

1. Prepare the pan: Line an 8 by 8–inch baking dish with aluminum foil so that it extends up the sides and over the edges of the pan. Spray the foil with cooking spray.

2. ***Make the crust:*** In a food processor, process the crackers into fine crumbles. Add the melted coconut oil and process again to combine. Pour the crumbs into the prepared pan and press down very firmly with your hands or a sheet of wax paper.

3. ***Make the filling:*** Combine the cashews, coconut milk, lime juice, honey, and coconut oil in a food processor and process until very smooth and creamy, scraping down the sides with a rubber spatula a couple of times (this will take about 5 minutes), or, for creamiest results, use a high-speed blender. Add the lime zest and pulse to combine it well. Spread the filling evenly over the crust.

4. Place the pan in the freezer and freeze until firm, about 2 hours.

5. Lift the cheesecake from the pan using the extended foil edges and place on a cutting board. Slide the foil out from under the cheesecake, cut the cheesecake into squares (a serrated knife works best), and pop into a freezer container or freezer bags.

6. Store in the freezer, remove 30 minutes before serving, and eat while still partially frozen.

A Coconut a Day Keeps the Doctor Away?

Extra-virgin olive oil is my go-to oil for most recipes, as it's heart-healthy, readily available, and affordable. But coconut oil is also worth exploring in savory dishes and particularly in dairy-free desserts as an alternative to cream or butter.

Coconut oil's fat is a unique type of saturated fat composed of medium-chain triglycerides, which are different from those found in meat and other vegetable oils; they possess anti-inflammatory and antioxidant properties, making coconut oil potentially heart-protective. Traditional people—from Southeast Asia to coastal Africa—have based their diets on coconut oil with relatively low incidence of heart disease (as coconut and other traditional foods were replaced with processed Western foods, heart disease started to appear more widely).

In South America they even say, "A coconut a day keeps the doctor away." And as a quick aside, coconut oil happens to be a great skin moisturizer to boot.

Berry Vanilla Granita

MAKES ABOUT 1 QUART

Here's a frozen dessert that's super-simple to put together, no ice cream maker required! Granita is a type of Italian frozen dessert somewhere between ices and sorbet and typically based on fruit, water, and sugar. Here we'll swap in honey for the white sugar and load our granita with antioxidant-rich berries for a satisfying and good-for-you summer snack. A scoop of Greek yogurt would be a welcome topping.

+ 1 quart fresh or thawed frozen raspberries, strawberries, or blackberries
+ 2 tablespoons fresh lemon juice
+ 1½ cups water
+ 2/3 cup light liquid honey, such as orange blossom or clover, or to taste
+ 1½ teaspoons pure vanilla extract
+ Pinch of salt

1. Combine the berries and lemon juice in a food processor and process until smooth. Transfer to a bowl, add the water, honey, vanilla, and salt, and whisk to dissolve the honey.

2. Pour the mixture into a 9-inch-square baking dish and place it in the freezer. Freeze until icy around the edges, about 30 minutes. Using a fork, stir the icy parts into the middle of the pan. Continue freezing

Continues ▶

and stirring the edges into the center every 20 minutes or so for about 3 hours, until the granita is almost completely frozen and the texture is similar to shaved ice. To serve, scrape the surface of the granita with a fork to create shaved ice crystals.

3. Scoop into dessert glasses and serve.

Frozen Yogurt Pops

SERVES 1

I'm generally a believer in plain yogurt, except when it comes to dessert. Most fruity yogurts are fairly high in sugar, so the best way to serve them is for dessert. Here's an effortless way to turn little containers of yogurt into fro-yo pops.

+ 1 small container yogurt, any flavor

1. Open the yogurt container and stir it if there's fruit at the bottom.
2. Place in the freezer for 10 to 15 minutes, then gently insert a wooden ice pop stick into the center.
3. Place back in the freezer for at least 3 hours, until frozen solid. To unmold, briefly dip the bottom of the container into a bowl of warm water, slip the yogurt pop out of the container, and serve.

LABEL 411

The Real Scoop on Frozen Desserts

Ice cream and frozen yogurt are once-in-a-while treats. (Don't worry—I'd never ask you to banish them from your life!) When you do indulge, go for the real thing—brands based on genuine dairy with no high-fructose corn syrup, preservatives, or artificial colors added. Pass on low-sugar options if it means an artificial sweetener is part of the picture. When you enjoy a small serving (about 1/2 cup) of good old-fashioned ice cream, you'll likely be satisfied and less likely to polish off the pint!

Tropical Chocolate Ice Cream

SERVES 2

Bananas are creamy dessert material, and since everything tastes better with chocolate, I've joined the two ingredients to make this satisfying frozen treat. Keep multiple bananas on hand in the freezer for whenever the ice cream craving hits.

+ 2 bananas, peeled, cut into chunks, and frozen
+ 2 to 3 tablespoons unsweetened cocoa powder, to taste
+ 1/2 teaspoon pure vanilla extract
+ About 3 tablespoons unsweetened coconut milk (not cream of coconut), almond milk, or other type of milk (just enough to get the ingredients moving in the food processor)
+ Optional toppings: fresh berries, unsweetened shredded coconut, cacao nibs

1. In a food processor, combine all the ingredients and process until smooth, scraping the sides of the machine with a rubber spatula two or three times, as needed.
2. Spoon into bowls and serve immediately, with your choice of toppings, if using.

Variation:

Tropical Chocolate Berry Ice Cream: Add a handful of frozen raspberries, strawberries, or cherries to the mix.